To Janet Blonder —
Best Wishes —
Hugh Mullen
11/2/83

VITAL SIGNS

Also by Fitzhugh Mullan

WHITE COAT, CLENCHED FIST:
THE POLITICAL EDUCATION OF AN
AMERICAN PHYSICIAN

VITAL SIGNS

A Young Doctor's Struggle
with Cancer

FITZHUGH MULLAN, M.D.

Farrar · Straus · Giroux

NEW YORK

Copyright © 1975, 1983 by Fitzhugh Mullan, M.D.

All rights reserved

Third Printing, 1983

Printed in the United States of America

Published simultaneously in Canada
by McGraw-Hill Ryerson Ltd., Toronto

Designed by Tere LoPrete

The four lines from the poem "To an Athlete Dying Young" on
p. 10 are from "A Shropshire Lad"—Authorized Edition—from
The Collected Poems of A. E. Housman. Copyright © 1939, 1940,
1965 by Holt, Rinehart and Winston. Copyright © 1967, 1968 by
Robert E. Symons. Reprinted by permission of Holt, Rinehart and
Winston, Publishers

Library of Congress Cataloging in Publication Data

Mullan, Fitzhugh.
    Vital signs.

      1. Chest—Cancer—Patients—United States—Biography.
2. Physicians—United States—Biography. 3. Mullan,
Fitzhugh. I. Title.
RC280.C5M84 1983   616.99'4'00924 [B]   82–15641

Certain of the persons mentioned in this book are referred to by
fictional names in order to insure that their identities remain
concealed

For my mother and father,
Mariquita and Hugh Mullan,
and my aunt,
Patricia MacManus

CONTENTS

Introduction	*ix*
Getting Sick	*3*
The Siege	*27*
Caitlin	*78*
Recalled	*100*
Revival	*141*
Taking Stock	*182*

INTRODUCTION

When at the age of thirty-two I discovered a mass deep within my chest that was most likely cancer, I had trouble understanding. I couldn't grasp what it meant for me or foretold for my family. I am a physician and I have seen illness of all sorts in people of all ages, but it was difficult to translate that into personal terms. Since I hadn't felt sick, the diagnosis seemed, at first, a total abstraction. I awoke one morning feeling as I always had, only to find myself declared a cancer patient by sundown. No amount of medical training and exposure could prepare me for so sudden and drastic an alteration in self-perception.

Fear and depression ganged up on me quickly, attacking by fits and starts during the first days of my new knowledge. Against them I had my strength and apparent good health, assets that I took for granted at the time but which I came to treasure and remember with nostalgia in the months to come. Since I was in no pain or physical distress, it was far easier to intellectualize the disease in that early stage than it would be later on. I now look back on those days as a period of innocence—an Indian summer before a winter whose grimness and anguish I could not possibly conceive. Scalpels had yet to cut my tissues, drugs to poison my cells, and radiation to scald my innards.

One particular incident from that period has stayed very much with me. In some ways, it is an example of my naïveté; in others, it is as prescient as any thought that I had at the time. Phil Spitzer is a good friend and my literary agent. When he heard about my condition he called immediately. He was upset and our conversation was halting. Still prior to my first hospitalization and still at a point when I could objectify the lump in my chest, I found myself working hard to cheer him up. "Look, Phil," I argued, "it's not so bad. Look at it this way. At the least we'll get a book out of it. I'll have some story to tell. Right?" Phil was unmoved. "Sure. Sure," he answered. I came away from our talk appreciative of his concern but a bit baffled that he didn't seem to grasp the beauty of the medico-journalistic scoop that had come our way. Phil, my agent, of all people, should be able to see the serendipity of a doctor-writer getting sick.

He didn't. He viewed me as a friend with a catastrophe on the way rather than a client with a clever angle for a book. To Phil any possible benefit that might emerge from the unfolding events was eclipsed by the horror of the events themselves. Skip the book, he seemed to be saying. Skip the book and stay with us. Don't put yourself through it. It can't be worth it.

Many times over the months that followed I reflected on that conversation and our differing perceptions. Amidst pain and fear and death wishes, I wondered how I ever could have been so frivolous, so misguided as to think that there would be *any* redeeming features of what was about to happen to me. I felt foolish that I, the doctor, had to be told by Phil, the man of letters, that sickness is terrible. The gravity with which he approached the situation proved to be appropriate, whereas my levity was a simple denial of a calamitous reality. In many ways the experiences to come were so painful I couldn't write about them and so embittering that I didn't want to. There was no serendipity, indeed nothing positive of any sort attached to my cancer. It was grim, brutal, and something to forget.

When I entered the hospital, however, my parents gave me a dictating machine, urging me to keep some sort of record of my feelings and the events. They were more interested in having a remembrance for themselves and the family than they were in promoting anything formally literary. I decided to use the machine from time to time—at first from a sense of duty (I should use it because it was such a nice gift) and later on from a greater sense of personal urgency. I came to want to tell the story, partly to leave something behind if I died and partly because it helped relieve my anger at my condition. With the aid of that recorder I developed a growing folder of reflections over the next three years—a collection of thoughts that gave credence to my original suggestion to Phil, that a book might come, after all, from my war with cancer.

Many months after my initial diagnosis, as I began to recover and life without pervasive illness once again became a reality for me, the desire to write about what had happened to me emerged strongly. My sense of what I was about, though, was different from what it had been when Phil and I had first talked. It was less the journalist in me that was itching to get out than it was the fellow traveler—the companion and soul-mate of millions of other people and families who were dueling with cancer. I had survived my illness and had discovered that there was much that I wanted to share with others who were going through it. That was a new perspective for me, one that I could not have appreciated before being sick but one that gave a new dimension to my urge to write.

As I started to think seriously about telling my story, other aspects of my experience came to mind. Sooner or later all doctors become patients, a role change that is never easy, although it does provide insights that are not learned in medical school. My time came sooner. It came early in my career and, strangely, in my own hands—I made my own diagnosis. In the aftermath of that diagnosis I learned a great deal that is not to be found in medical textbooks. My experiences made me both a greater admirer and a harsher critic of my profession and intensified my desire to describe what happened for the benefit of doctors and patients.

I was young for a cancer patient. I knew virtually no one my age who was sick, let alone had cancer. I discovered this to be a handicap at the time of my first hospitalization, since I had few role models and no one with whom to compare notes or lick wounds. After leaving the hospital I was called on to catch up with life in mid-race. I didn't return to a retirement village or a senior citizens' community. I rejoined a wife and a growing family of my own as well as an ongoing career as a physician. I reentered an athletic world, a business world, a sexual world.

Over the months I heard stories about other young people with cancer and the atypical and difficult situations they encountered. A young woman, a nurse, who had had Hodgkin's disease, told me of the chilling effect disclosure of her illness had on the amorous interest of doctors she dated. The dialogue she described ran like this: "That little scar on your neck, a biopsy?" "Yes." Pause. "Everything turn out all right?" "No. Actually it didn't." Long pause. "Gee. Too bad." The flirtation would end abruptly at that point.

The unlikely calamities, the mean quirks that befall young people with cancer surprised even me as I learned of them. I discovered a horrible family imbroglio concerning a woman in her thirties and her mother three decades older. The two were dying simultaneously of cancer, each furious with the other for stealing her moment of uncompromised love and attention. The two virtually asked their family to take sides as to which of them was more deserving of compassion. The family, needless to say, was in agony over the illnesses and their circumstance.

A friend confided to me the story of his marriage when he was in his early twenties. His wife developed a small skin growth that, to everyone's astonishment, proved to be a metastasis from a malignant lymphoma growing within her. Several more skin lesions occurred and only minimal therapy was attempted on the presumption that the disease was widespread and untreatable. They waited and watched and tried to live as well as they could. Nothing happened. The tension was tremendous. In spite of the ghost of cancer that went everywhere with them, they went ahead bravely and had a child. Still nothing happened. After two years the tension proved too great. The woman ran away, seeking solace in drugs and the counterculture, leaving my friend to raise their child alone. He found his wife again some years later. She was cancer-free and sane, but she never came home.

As I struggled with these stories and my own, I came to believe that the problems of young people with cancer were more complex and far less explored than I had ever realized. This made me the more eager to share my experiences in the hope that they would be helpful to other young adults facing cancer or similar life-altering crises.

Introduction

Transforming a folder of notes taken over three years into a coherent story did not prove to be an easy task. I found it especially difficult for reasons I have come to appreciate only in retrospect. The role of autobiographer is a hard one. While it requires the precision and discipline of all writing, it enjoys neither the distance of the historian or the biographer nor the dramatic liberties of the novelist. Particularly difficult is the balance between material that is, of necessity, intimate and the need for some sort of objectivity. And labor I would to give the story a sense of objectivity. Objectivity! I was still very much in the shadow of my cancer, reminded almost hourly by one discomfort or another that at the very least I was physically and statistically still within its reach. How objective could I be? How much of my rage at the illness and its tentacles could I have resolved?

Not much.

Yet there is a right time to write. Early on I didn't want to write anything about what had happened. I didn't want to remember it, rehash it, or relive it in any way. Even three years after the worst of it, listening to tapes of people I recorded or rereading my transcribed notes, I became terribly anxious and unsure of my resolve to write. The passage of time made the events less immediate, and more objectivity—or, at least, dispassion—became possible. Yet the vividness of the story started to fade as well, which is not good for the reporter. So I began to work my small pile of observations into a more thoughtful and coherent commentary, trying as hard as I could to look beyond my anger and my still-present bitterness.

As I wrote, a new problem emerged—the survivor's conundrum. Over the years many writers—indeed, many artists—knowing they were terminally ill, have bent their skills to some final work, a statement that often involves the disease. The dying autobiographer has a legitimately Olympian claim—or as legitimate as a human ever has. The surviving autobiographer has a different point of purchase, one that, whatever its merits, does not command the finality and sense of aloofness that the true death statement does. The vision is tempered by the passion and subjectivity that I have described as well as a very obvious and important ongoing investment in life. Comments about other people and about oneself remain with the survivor while they don't trouble the deceased writer. How does one write about his doctors when some of them are still treating him? How does the survivor treat his family and friends when he is living and working among them? Most difficult, how does one dissect oneself before a public that is still very much with him?

Vital Signs is a living testament and not a parting shot. Phil was right that the disease was terrible but I wasn't wrong that it would be worth telling about. And the telling of that tale makes the entire event a little more acceptable to me. It records the reality of what I experienced. It shares the trials and joys of what happened with friends and family who watched from the near distance. It tells—and will tell—my children something about me. And to the many whose lives have been disrupted by cancer, it extends a hand—a gesture of friendship, kinship, and hope.

To Judy, my wife, I owe a special word of thanks. Not only did she live with me through every up and down of the disease but she also widowed herself to a typewriter for long periods of time while I wrote the story. That is double jeopardy and this is double thanks and then some. My friend and typist Pauline Lieberman likewise suffered with us through the episodes I describe and then devotedly transcribed them. My special appreciation goes to her as well.

Garrett Park, Maryland
November 1982

VITAL SIGNS

CHAPTER

I

Getting Sick

The mother of the squalling one-year-old met me in the emergency room. The infant had been running a fever for a week and was eating poorly and had a cough. I ordered a chest X-ray, and since I wanted to read it myself, I took the mother and child to the X-ray unit. While I waited for the film to be shot I thought of getting a chest X-ray for myself. For the previous three months I had suffered occasional pain in my chest that awoke me at night. For three weeks following an episode of flu, I had been coughing. The X-ray technician was happy to oblige me, and within minutes I was standing in front of the developing machine waiting for two sets of X-rays—the child's and my own.

The child's X-ray revealed a tiny well-formed chest with a definitive right middle lobe infiltrate. I felt satisfied because I had made the correct diagnosis and because I had something definite to treat in this ill child—a pneumonia that would respond promptly to antibiotics.

Before I had finished looking at the baby's films mine came sliding out. I had taken only a single view of my chest, assuming I would find nothing. I stuffed the plastic rectangle under the lip of the viewing box and peered into my own chest. My first glance told me that something was very wrong. To the right of the heart and confluent with its border was a fluffy white density that extended into all lobes of the right lung. It was the size of a grapefruit, but on the X-ray looked like a hazy cauliflower.

The physician in me responded first and I instinctively looked at the grim information on the viewing box as a clinician. This was an unusual finding, a fascinating X-ray, I said to myself. There are a number of possibilities that will have to be considered. I took the two sets of films to the radiologists down the hall. I enjoyed bringing positive X-rays to the specialists to show them I knew what I was doing and because I usually learned something as well. This trip was no exception. I still had not focused on the fact that the pathology I was going to display was my own.

They confirmed the child's pneumonia and put my film on the view box. When I told them it was me, there was an immediate change in their casual manner. They weighed their words carefully as they examined the radiograph and awkwardly asked me a few questions. The changed demeanor of these friends of mine cut through my clinical dispassion and raised the first red flag in my mind. I felt my initial fear.

They ordered a lateral view, which confirmed a large mass in the center of my chest. "The last one of these we saw was a dermoid," said one radiologist to the other. "It was shelled out with no problem." His comment disturbed me by what it obviously omitted —that most of "these" do not end up as "no problem." Most of these are malignancies, and all of them are dangerous.

By now I was beginning to come to grips with what was happening. That pint-sized cauliflower that I had so recently discovered on a piece of celluloid was in fact a tumor—a cancer. It was living quietly deep within *my* body. Though I had no knowledge at that point of what kind of cancer it was, its strategic location suggested that it could bring my life to an end at any time. In a space of five minutes it had come out of nowhere to become the focal point of my life, or perhaps the focal point of the rest of my life.

I wrote a penicillin prescription for the infant with pneumonia, gave the mother a few instructions, and went to the changing room to get into a hospital gown. The radiologist wanted to take X-rays of my abdomen. The smock he gave me was absurdly short and as I padded down the corridor in my stocking feet with my knees showing I suddenly understood that I was a patient.

I was thirty-two years old at the time, working for the U.S. Public Health Service as a physician at a community clinic in the *barrio* of Santa Fe. My wife, Judy, and I had lived in Santa Fe for three years and had come to love New Mexico. We had a three-year-old daughter, Meghan. All of us had been in good health and both Judy's parents and mine were alive and well. Illness had not been part of our life in any way. I suppose I thought that someday one or another of us would become sick and perhaps die but, at least for me and for Judy and Meghan, that seemed quite remote. Illness—asthma, cystic fibrosis, diabetes mellitus, and cancer—happened elsewhere. The worst that happened to us was colds, diarrhea, and rashes.

As I climbed onto the cold, metallic X-ray table I had reason and time to think about this. The X-ray that the radiologist had scheduled for me was an intravenous pyelogram, which required sequential views of my kidneys over a half-hour period. During that time I was not to leave the table. Lying on that hospital slab, staring at the maze of electronic equipment over my head on that March morning in 1975, I felt alone and in agony, desperate to talk to someone —the physician I had picked to consult, my wife, my parents, anyone. I was bursting to share the calamity. But all I could do was lie there with my eyes helplessly scanning the gadgetry around the room, looking for some safe harbor from the anxiety that suddenly inundated me.

6

The kidney films proved normal. A tiny victory. I dressed and found a phone to call Judy. As a secretary went to find her I mused unhappily about what was about to befall her. "Hi, Fitz. What is it?" she said cheerily when she came to the phone. I started to cry. I hung on the wall phone in the hospital corridor hoping that no one would see me sobbing, trying to explain to my wife that I had a thing in my chest that surely meant our lives were drastically changed. "Stay there," she told me. "I'll be right over." She arrived quickly and together we took the X-rays to a chest specialist. We sat in his office holding hands, waiting to present my case for the first time, something I was to do frequently in the weeks to come. When he looked at the films he agreed that tumor was the inescapable diagnosis. The only way to be sure of the type of tumor was to perform a biopsy. This would have to be done under general anesthesia through an incision in the lower neck that would allow the surgeon to gently enter the mediastinum, the area between the lungs and around the heart which houses a host of vital structures. The tumor was growing among them and would have to be approached and biopsied through a long instrument, a procedure called mediastinoscopy. We left his office and walked out into the New Mexico noonday sun in a daze.

Judy and I made things better that afternoon with a time-honored medicinal, rum and Coke. We did not attempt to explain to Meghan what was happening. Several good friends spent the evening with us, sharing the rum.

Since I was a member of the Public Health Service, I was entitled to treatment at any military facility. I decided to go to Washington, D.C., which had the heaviest concentration of large military hospitals. Also, my parents lived in Washington and this gave us a base of operation. Barely twenty-four hours after my visit to the X-ray unit I left Santa Fe to start the flight East. Judy and Meghan were staying behind for the moment; they drove me to the airport in Albuquerque, a pretty hour-and-a-half trip through classic New Mexico scenery. I gazed out fondly at the distant craggy mountains and the buttes and bluffs of the high mountain desert.

As the plane circled around the Sandia Mountains and climbed to the east I felt an ache of nostalgia. The brown plains below with their Indian and Spanish heritage had become my home. I didn't know if I would ever see them again. I looked around at the other passengers on the flight and wondered what sundry business and social events were carrying them across the country. Perhaps someone else on board had a malignancy and was traveling to a medical center for treatment. Certainly it wasn't inconceivable. I found myself wishing that I could know who that person was so that we could sit together and share our extraordinary bond.

My parents and brother and sister met me at the

airport when I arrived. It was an emotional moment for us all. As I walked down the aseptic tube from the plane to the airport I knew what they must be thinking. What would their son look like, now that he bore a dangerous warrant within him? Would I look different? Would I look thinner, grayer, older? I did not feel one bit different than before my discovery and I was sure my looks had not changed at all. As I turned into the waiting room I was intent on showing them there was nothing to worry about. We clasped one another and they wanted to carry my bag and my coat. I refused. They acquiesced gracefully, for, devastated though I know they were, they were determined to be supportive, evenhanded, and flexible from that first night on.

During the next three or four days I lived in a kind of limbo between doctor and patient. I discussed my options with several private consultants and a number of military physicians. At each visit I presented my case history and my X-rays simply and dispassionately. In fact, I discovered, to my surprise, that I liked presenting my case. It felt appropriate and safe when I discussed my chest growth from a clinical point of view. The familiar role kept my fear at bay and allowed me some comfort in spite of the life-shattering diagnoses we invariably discussed. As long as I could play doctor to my disease, I learned, I could at least partially protect myself from the anxiety and feelings of helplessness that accompanied my new status.

Even death did not seem frightening to me at this

stage. If it were to happen, I remember thinking, at least I had not lived badly. At thirty-two my glass was half full. In later weeks I would come to think of my glass as half empty, and the prospect of death became awesome and infuriating. I reread a poem I remembered from high school—A.E. Housman's "To an Athlete Dying Young." The verses suggest that it is not at all bad to die a youthful death, strong, honored, and well remembered.

> Now you will not swell the rout
> Of lads that wore their honours out,
> Runners whom renown outran
> And the name died before the man.

The poem offered a comforting rationale for the worst possible outcome of my chest problem.

Four days after my trip, Judy and Meghan flew East and joined my encampment at Mom and Dad's house. Judy accompanied me on a visit to the headquarters of the Public Health Service to discuss our situation with the director of the Medical Branch. We wanted to review our insurance coverage and entitlements depending upon the outcome of the impending surgery. A popular tune playing quietly on a radio in the background suddenly overwhelmed us. Its melody was familiar and engaging, but the song, "Seasons in the Sun," had never meant anything to us before. It describes the relationship between two young friends, one of whom is dying. Gradually, wordlessly, we both began to cry. Then, with difficulty, we blotted our tears and tried to laugh a little about how maudlin we had become.

The doctors all agreed that diagnostic mediastinoscopy was the next step. Without a tissue diagnosis no one could discuss treatment or prognosis. I chose the National Naval Medical Center in Bethesda since it had a good reputation in surgery and I liked the doctors I met there. The hospital is an impressive one set on an attractive campus across the street from the National Institutes of Health and dominated by "The Tower"—an eighteen-story building rising above the Maryland countryside. I was admitted to the thoracic surgery service on the ninth floor—so-called Tower Nine.

Although the U.S. Public Health Service is technically a uniformed service run in parallel with the armed forces, it in fact functions in a far more informal manner. As a community-based physician in New Mexico, I neither wore nor owned a uniform. Although I had a military rank, I had to pause to remember what it was. The Naval Hospital, I knew, was going to be a different sort of experience for me and I was curious as to what it was going to be like.

When I checked into the hospital I registered at the admissions office. While I was waiting for my paperwork to be completed, a young black man in standard Navy issue, bathrobe and pajamas, approached, looking me up and down. "Are you a dependent?" he asked.

At first I wasn't sure what he meant. Then it dawned on me that something about my demeanor suggested to him that I wasn't military myself and that, instead, I must be the husband of a woman in the military. "No, I'm not a dependent," I answered.

"Well then, what are you?"

I wasn't quite sure what to respond, but I knew I was being checked out by the Navy. A number of possible answers flashed through my mind and I chose the one that seemed the most martial. "I'm an officer," I said.

"You're an officer? With all that hair?" I don't have all that much hair, I thought. It covered the tops of my ears and curled a little around the back of my neck. "What kind of service are you in, anyway?"

I laughed and explained that I was in the Public Health Service, which was not a standard military service as far as dress and discipline went. He looked long and hard at me, apparently finding it difficult to believe that I had any kind of military status. At length, mollified, he said, "I thought you was awful big to be a dependent." His criticism was gentle and, since I felt comfortable enough in the Navy environment, it didn't bother me. Had it not been for the grimness of the business at hand, I think I would have enjoyed this first opportunity to observe military life from the inside.

Less than a week after my visit to the X-ray unit with the one-year-old with pneumonia, I was ensconced on Tower Nine. It was a pleasant place, well staffed with nurses and hospital corpsmen. In fact, I found it amusing and instructive to experience the hospital from the other side after so many years of doctoring. I chuckled as I lay in bed while the surgeons made their early rounds. Navy corpsmen brought me my meals and looked after my needs and I enjoyed the attention of the nurses.

My first discomfort as a patient came when the surgeon who was to operate on me passed a bronchoscope (a hose-like tube) down my windpipe to be sure that my bronchi had not been obstructed by the tumor. A bedside bronchoscopy with a fiberoptic scope is a neat, space-age procedure, but its side effects include choking, tearing, and a residual sore throat. The surgeon stopped partway through the exam, bent the flexible tube 180 degrees, and let me peer into my right main-stem bronchus, where I could see the tumor partially compressing the bronchus. For a crazy, order-defying moment I was doctor and patient all at once.

But my true dependency as a patient was quickly impressed upon me. Two mornings in a row, after fasting from midnight and preparing myself as well as I could psychologically, my surgery was canceled. Twice the nurse came and told me that the surgeons had called to say emergencies had come up. Twice I had to call Judy and tell her to change plans. Twice I had to explain to myself that it would *not* be over by sundown and that the shadow that threatened to destroy my life was still nameless.

The cancellations shattered my defenses and sent me into a deep depression. By then it was clear to me that my disease and my life were out of my hands. I could make a good case presentation, discuss the differential diagnosis, or even look down my own bronchoscope, but I could not control the real decisions and actions concerning my disease. Due to the delays my surgeon was changed. I was now slated to be operated on by Dr. Mitchell Mills, Chief of the Thoracic Surgery Service. Fiftyish and unassuming, Mills was a Navy captain and, as I later learned, the architect of an unusual and genteel surgical service. He was the unquestioned boss of Tower Nine and over subsequent months he became a friend and counselor.

By the third morning I was limp. I had successfully—if briefly—turned my depression into relaxation. I had decided that since none of the decisions were mine, none of the trials or worries were mine either. I was determined to doze through the preoperative period. That resolve was made easier by the fact that I was the first case scheduled and the preoperative routine started for me at 5 a.m. with yet another trip to the shower room with surgical soap to scrub my neck and chest. At this point my skin was raw from preparation. My showers had assumed a ceremonial quality.

As a final reminder of my complete subservience to the system, I was stripped bare, placed on a rolling stretcher, covered with a thin sheet, and wheeled through the halls of the hospital to the surgical suite. My glasses had been left neatly on my bedside table, so everything appeared fuzzy as I whizzed by on my way to the surgical never-never land. Nonetheless, the thought of riding in a public elevator stark naked, protected only by a drafty sheet, made me anxious. It epitomized my vulnerability. At 6:30 in the morning the elevator proved to be empty and the halls relatively unpopulated, so I made the best of the voyage and experienced no embarrassment.

When we arrived in the surgical area I was parked in what proved to be the recovery room alongside a number of other supine sheet-clad figures. Though I did no checking, I presumed that they also had left their pajamas in their rooms. As far as I could tell without my glasses, we were men and women, large and small, and our ranks continued to swell until the recovery room was fairly packed. We were surely an unusual congregation, nude, pensive, and silent. Many of us were premedicated with a variety of drugs to induce relaxation. I had declined any, fearing perhaps any more loss of control than I had already experienced. In any event, I managed to feel relaxed despite the strange circumstances and the impending event. I shut my eyes and without benefit of warmth or pillow dozed comfortably. At one point during the wait I was awakened by an attendant who pointed out that the sheet had slipped and my numb behind was exposed. He asked me rather aseptically to cover it. His concern seemed to be about germs rather than sex, suggesting that I was more patient than person—an attitude I would come to know well. I obliged and dozed off again.

After a time the orderly returned, checked my bracelet and chart, and wheeled me into the operating room. Being "prepped" for surgery is a unique human experience. It is both an egotist's dream and a procedure uncannily like the preparation of a human sacrifice. In the absolute inner temple of the hospital I was assisted onto the draped altar. My sheet was removed and orderlies bathed and rebathed the point of entry. Anesthesiologists busied themselves with my arms, running intravenous fluids into one and strapping tools to the other. Skilled nurses counted and arranged the soon-to-be-bloodied instruments on trays at the periphery of the room. The surgeons strolled in and out chatting in muted, important tones, haggling quietly over the fine points on the X-rays on illuminated wall boxes, all the time scrubbing their hands and arms with time-honored ritual diligence. It was a bizarre luxury to lie there smugly with the knowledge that all of this was being done for me and that I would have no assignment or responsibility in the unfolding events except to lie back and accept.

Little by little the anesthesiologist took over, strapping a mask to my face and explaining procedures to me one after another. First atropine was given painlessly through the IV. He promised me I would feel my heart beat harder and, in thirty seconds, I did. Next there was the curare, a muscle paralyzer borrowed by the surgeons from South American Indians. It is used to immobilize the muscles of respiration in cases where the patient is to be intubated for the purpose of artificial breathing. If the patient cannot fight the tube passed down the throat, the process is far more effective. I would feel weak, he told me, when he gave a test dose of curare, and perhaps I would see double, since the ocular muscles are among the most sensitive. I felt relaxed and even confident. I nodded assent. I was glad *I* didn't have to worry about the appropriate dose of curare. Slowly the surgical lights overhead did double and then they faded out.

The operation was under way.

In some ways death is more understandable an experience than anesthesia. There is something terminal, definitive, and relatively fathomable about death. Anesthesia, on the contrary, invites belief in a state where the mind disappears while the body is cut apart and manipulated, only to return oblivious to the events that have occurred. On its face anesthesia is implausible. I had observed this chain of events many times and participated in it. Yet, approached personally, it seemed more unlikely than ever.

Having gone under and returned, I can offer no clarification of the seeming improbability of anesthesia. As things turned out, the surgical procedure went awry and my body had to be torn open. Twice

I came perilously close to death—events that involved Dr. Mills, Judy, my family, and a host of other people. These were the most critical events of my life. I slumbered through them, effectively and unfathomably absent from their reality or their recollection. Their occurrence distressed everybody involved with them as they happened except for me.

My first consciousness came in darkness with muffled noises in the distance. Clumsily my mind began to palpate the undifferentiated sensations that were beginning to move within it. I remembered that I was in the hospital and had just had an operation, but I was unable to move any part of my body. I could not open my eyes or wiggle my fingertips. In fact, I was unable to let the outside world know that I was awake.

Then I recalled the curare, the last thing I had focused on before the operation. The continued presence of paralytic curare in my veins made some kind of sense to me and was comforting. I don't know how long that state of affairs went on and I am sure that my mind was less lucid than I felt it was. I dozed back into a semi-anesthetized sleep. I don't remember any anxiety associated with my first thoughts, but I was perplexed and annoyed not to be able to contact anyone or anything. It is a strange sensation not to be able to open your eyelids. It seemed unreasonable to me that I could not at least do that.

When I heard the unmistakable rhythmic wheeze of a respirator somewhere near me, I understood better what was happening. It was my respirator and it was breathing for me. The curare had not been randomly administered, but was part of a treatment plan that included a machine to do my breathing. Slowly I became aware of the tube in my throat and my chest rising and falling with the mechanical gasping. How often I had been on the other end of a respirator. It amused me to lie there the patient of a machine, paralyzed supplicant to the science I had so often practiced. I drifted back into unconsciousness.

Eventually in this timeless state I began to move a little and to be able to open my eyes. I don't remember whom I recognized first. Judy, Mom, Dad, and Dr. Mills all visited me. My only way to communicate with them was by squeezing their hands, since my mouth and throat were rammed full of gadgetry. Their squeezes and warm smiles were incredibly important to me. I began to focus on the quantities of tape on my chest and I realized that I was in the intensive care unit rather than the recovery room. All of this seemed to add up to much more serious an operative procedure than the simple mediastinal biopsy for which I had been scheduled.

Gradually I became able to move my index finger well enough to write a simple word of inquiry on the palms of outstretched hands. "Why?" I inquired of Mom—meaning why all the paraphernalia. The operation had been complicated, she told me. "When?" I asked Judy. It proved to be Friday evening, the end of the same long day that had begun with the stretcher trip through the hospital corridors—Good Friday, 1975, as we were to reflect frequently afterward.

When I was fully awake Dr. Mills explained to me gently what had happened. The biopsy had bled, necessitating an emergency thoracotomy—a chest-splitting procedure that opens the thorax down the front and around under the breast to the back. In my case, it was done on a crash basis to get sufficient exposure to stem the flow of blood. That had been a difficult and long procedure but, once having stopped the bleeding, they had decided to remove as much of the tumor as possible since it lay exposed before them. He estimated they had taken 60 percent of it. The pathologists had identified the tumor as a seminoma, an unusual tumor occasionally found in the chest, but one that was amenable to treatment and potential cure. Dr. Mills was direct and reassuring, and I drifted back into my narcotized sleep with a sense that cure was a possibility.

Sensibly, Dr. Mills had given me only a sketch of the events of that day. As I found out later, the tumor was massive and had grown around and through a number of vital structures in the mediastinum, including the superior vena cava, the innominate vein, a number of key nerves, the pericardium, and the right lung. Through the mediastinoscope it had been difficult to tell what was tumor and what was not. The innominate vein, which carries quantities of blood from the upper body back to the heart, was lurking just beneath the tissue chosen for the biopsy. After the bite was taken it poured forth its contents, obscuring the field and blinding the mediastinoscope. The surgeons had to work quickly, splitting my sternum and extending the incision across my right breast and up under my right armpit in order to open the chest far enough to get at the bleeding. They started to pour blood into me immediately and more was ordered hastily from the blood bank. In all it took seven units, more than half my original circulating volume, to replace the loss.

At length the bleeding was controlled, but there was little time for rest, since by stages the surgeons realized my pulse was becoming rapid and shallow and my blood pressure was falling. After a quick inspection of the surgical field they discovered I was suffering cardiac tamponade. Blood had leaked down inside the pericardium, the covering of the heart, and it was slowly, lethally welling up. The pericardium is a tough tissue and does not expand significantly under pressure. The effect of the internal blood flow, then, was to strangle the heart and prevent its beating, a fatal circumstance if it is not treated quickly. Recognizing the problem, Dr. Mills cut a window in the pericardium, relieving the pressure and allowing the heart to resume its normal volume and rhythm.

Having finally brought the situation under control and stabilized the bleeding and having received a tentative tissue diagnosis from the pathology lab, they took on the tumor. The more they could dig out, they reasoned, the more effective the subsequent therapies would be. They proceeded to do that and then closed the chest, leaving a variety of tubes and drains in place and maintaining my breathing on the ventilator.

Judy and my parents had assembled that morning in the waiting room outside the surgical suite. They had been told that the surgery would be completed shortly after 9 a.m. and that they would be able to visit with me within the hour and we would have a tissue diagnosis by noon. They arrived slowly, Judy first, then Mom. Dad and my sister Quita appeared a little later, followed eventually by my brother Tony. Sometime between nine and ten, Rob Hill, a Navy chaplain whom we had met the day before, came to tell them that there had been some complications and he would keep them informed. For the next six hours Chaplain Hill served as emissary from the operating table to the anxious group in the waiting room. Clad in a green surgical scrub suit, disposable mask flapping over his chest, taking stairs three at a time, he jogged back and forth between the surgeons and the family, describing the events in the operating room. He suggested that Judy contact her parents in Minneapolis and ask them to come to Washington immediately. He placed the call for her. On the advice of the surgeons, he asked his Catholic counterpart to give me last rites. The surgeons, understanding military benefits well, advised that procedures be initiated to have me retired immediately, since death benefits for retired officers are superior to those for active-duty officers. Chaplain Hill coordinated efforts to contact the appropriate people in the Public Health Service. Fortunately, as it turned out, the retirement couldn't be put through that quickly and I remained "on active duty."

The pain that my family suffered that Good Friday is impossible for me to appreciate. Relief came in midafternoon when they learned that my chest was being closed and that I would survive the operation. I am sure that the gentle hand squeezes in the ICU that evening were as meaningful for them as they were for me.

It was good to have the surgery behind me. I lay back (my only option really) and watched the dance of the ICU take place around me. My chest tubes were pumped regularly, blood gases were taken from my wrist, the respirator was slowly withdrawn, and coughing and deep-breathing therapies were instituted. I was grateful for the attention and skill of the Navy corpsmen and nurses who took care of me at all hours. The corpsmen, in particular, were a study in efficiency. There was one assigned to me at all times. I was his only patient and he spent virtually his entire shift caring for me. He knew his machinery, his cardiac monitors, his blood gas machine, his respirator, and he knew his patient, my problems, and the potential complications. Under the direction of the surgeons and with the backup of the nurses, three skillful young men ran my body for thirty-six hours and did a superlative job. Carefully they gave me my first postoperative bath, looked after my pain, and answered my questions about my condition. Aside from the gratitude I will always feel for their care, they were a case study in paramedical technology. With no more than high school diplomas behind them, these twenty-year-olds had been trained as crack human technicians. They brought the fruit of centuries of science to bear on my body. I was appreciative.

I found the occasional presence of the doctors welcome but insubstantial. As a physician, I knew the hours of anxiety that having a patient in the intensive care unit meant, always on guard, always worried. Now that I was a patient, however, the doctors' efforts seemed almost inconsequential. In the heat of the battle the doctor appeared as a general sitting on some distant hill. It was the people with me, running the machinery, who counted. In their skilled hands my life slowly flowed back. On the second postoperative day I returned to my room on Tower Nine.

In Santa Fe, I had worked at La Clínica de la Gente, the Clinic of the People. It was a community-governed medical practice housed in a former convent on the outskirts of Santa Fe. The Public Health Service supplied the medical staff, including me. La Clínica sponsored a basketball team in the Santa Fe City Men's League. Basketball had been an abiding love of mine since third grade. Our game was strictly street ball, a lot of one-on-one, rough under the boards, and good camaraderie. We held our own against such perennial City League stalwarts as PAC Plumbing, the State Pen, Music Villa, and the Public Service Company.

Early in March of 1975, two weeks before my fateful chest X-ray, we entered the City League tournament. On a sunny Sunday afternoon we played and won our first play-off game. In keeping with local tradition, Judy and Meghan came and sat in the stands and cheered. I played well and felt accomplished as only basketball could make me feel. After the game I completed the masculine ritual by accompanying my teammates to a local bar while Judy and Meghan went home. We went to a Chicano dive behind a shopping center off the main road to Albuquerque. We listened to mariachi music on the jukebox, recapitulated the game in Spanish and in English, and downed two pitchers of beer, a happy albeit broken-down version of "Miller Time."

I said goodbye to the team and got in my car to go home. It was about five o'clock on a Sunday afternoon. The sun was brilliant gold, illuminating Santa Fe and the Rio Grande Valley stretching to the west. With two beers and a basketball game under my belt I felt euphoric. I sped along Cerrillos Road and St. Michaels Drive looking at the businesses shut tight on Sunday. I climbed to the north past the scrub pinyon trees where the new St. Vincent's Hospital was to be built and looked straight ahead at the snowcapped Sangre de Cristo Mountains rising above the city. The Santa Fe ski basin was hidden in those mountains and would be just closing for the day. Packs of happy, sunburned skiers would be descending the narrow road down the mountain. They too must have felt the beauty of the day with winter passing and spring almost palpable. I turned down Santa Fe Avenue toward home, where I knew Judy was fixing dinner. It was a moment of exquisite happiness.

I could not possibly have had any inkling of the problems to come and yet that is what euphoria is all about. It ignores the possibility of catastrophe and unhappiness. It is a moment of freedom, a moment of perfect flight, that belies, discounts, forgets, and denies all other possibilities. In the time that followed that early March afternoon I thought frequently of that moment. I clung to its memory as proof that happiness exists. My body was to become a vessel of pain, nausea, depression, and despair. I clung to the memory of that golden twilight in the belief that bodies were made for something better than what I felt.

CHAPTER
2

The Siege

In the first days following surgery the full extent of my illness became clearer to me. No longer was I able to appear hearty and brave. In spite of the mental weight of the disease in the preoperative period, my body had continued to function unflinchingly with scarcely a hint of the problems inside. That was all changed after surgery. The post-thoracotomy patient is extremely sick regardless of the underlying diagnosis. My breastbone had been split, several ribs were cracked, my heart had been manipulated and was subject to failure, and my lungs had been literally manhandled. Pneumonia, fluid and electrolyte imbalance, congestive heart failure, internal bleeding, and infection were all possibilities. Superimposed on these threats was pain—pain caused by breathing, moving, and, above all, coughing.

Coughing, however, was a critical part of the therapy, to clear the lungs. In my first hours back on the ward I was given a "coughing pillow" by an affable nurse. She explained the principle carefully. The coughing pillow was a piece of heavy plywood mightily bandaged with gauze and tape. I was to clutch it to my breast when I coughed to avoid the sensation of splitting my chest open. I was to use it hourly during the coughing sessions that the corpsmen would initiate. The pillow, she claimed, would allow me to cough more deeply, thereby clearing my lungs more effectively. She was right, but the pain was terrible anyway. Wherever I went for the next three weeks I took my silly little pillow with me. It was a security blanket of a very functional sort.

Tower Nine staff had additional tricks to promote breathing. Foremost among them was a tabletop breathing instrument that took advantage of the human competitive instinct. Not unlike the "test your strength" contraption at a county fair, this machine invited the breather to move as much air as possible in a single breath. The results were measured on a gauge which protruded from the top of the machine. The exercise caused pulmonary expansion and frequently promoted coughing—an uncomfortable but effective series of events. I was awakened through the night to perform these pulmonary calisthenics.

Although pain and physical incapacity were the primary aspects of the postoperative period, the continued search for cancer was another uncomfortable ingredient. I underwent serial X-rays, multiple radio-isotope scans conducted by large machines that took pictures of my brain, my bones, my liver, my lungs—in short, my body from head to toe. Additionally, I had a bone marrow biopsy—a painful bite out of my hip bone—and frequent exams by specialists. These were all procedures that as a doctor I had ordered and observed before. Now I was being pushed down long corridors in a wheelchair with my coughing pillow, to have them performed on me, the patient. A strange experience. Pilots cannot become planes, I remember thinking, nor can auto mechanics change into carburetors. But here I am, the doctor, wheeling through the hospital with my IV dripping overhead on my way to have my bone marrow sampled. Weird. How weird!

It was also strange to regard my body with suspicion. It had always before served me well and, other than an occasional twinge of curiosity about my coronary arteries, I had never given much thought to the functioning or malfunctioning of my body's various parts. I assumed they would do a pretty good job and they did. The cancer in my chest destroyed all of that, absolutely and permanently. No longer was I confident of my body. It had failed me. Moreover, the failure was caused by the surreptitious enemy named cancer, a guerrilla fighter that called into question virtually all the rest of my being. Was it lurking elsewhere? Was there a fifth column in my liver, an insurrectionary cell in my brain, a malignant reinforcement in my belly? I could be sure of nothing.

Furthermore, the tumor was a seminoma, which is a cancer of testicular tissue that usually starts as a swelling in the scrotum of young men. I had experienced no such swelling and, although seminomas do arise spontaneously in the chest, the origin of mine was as yet uncertain. Had it really started in my chest or was it, in fact, an outpost established by a testicular death squad dispatched many months earlier from my groin? My reproductive cells—the very center of my private being—fell under suspicion. I felt betrayed by my body.

The battery of tests and examinations revealed no further evidence of malignancy. No one could be sure what would be the effects of the massive pot-stirring that had occurred on the operating table. It was concluded by Dr. Mills, in consultation with the other specialists, that radiation and chemotherapy should be started in mid-April, about two weeks after the surgery, when my chest had begun to heal.

That schedule, as it turned out, was suddenly moved ahead. At the end of the first week an eerie process began to take place. Almost imperceptibly at first, and then more pronouncedly, my upper body began to swell. My head felt like a stuffed cabbage. My eyes protruded ever so slightly and my cheeks puffed up. My mouth was dry and my vocal cords became hoarse and raspy. My arms started to swell, so that it was impossible to draw blood and I could no longer get my wedding ring on my finger. I was diagnosed as having the Superior Vena Caval Syndrome. The superior vena cava, the massive pipe that collects blood from the upper body and dumps it back into the heart, had been invaded and largely obliterated by the tumor. The surgery itself had caused swelling and bleeding in the area. The continued growth of the tumor as well as postsurgical swelling was precipitating the total blockage of that crucial vessel. The experience was terrifying. I understood the physiology of what was happening well enough to know that it was an ominous sign. Even without that precise knowledge, the sensation of a bloated head and grotesquely swollen hands—of being a balloon man—would have been acutely frightening.

The symptoms had emerged during the weekend, and late on Sunday afternoon it was decided that radiation therapy should be started on an emergency basis in an effort to stem the growth of the tumor. In my medical training I had spent almost no time with radiation therapy. As a topic, it had always depressed me, since, reasonably, I associated it with cancer. As I began to think about my own impending radiation treatment I realized that I harbored many prejudices against radiation therapists and their practices. I thought of the radiation therapists I had known in medical school as the most awkward, the most pallid, and the least attractive faculty members. It seemed to me that they were comfortable with slide rules and electronic consoles but not with people. They spent their working time in deep underground cells dug to house the dangerous machinery they drove. Radiation therapy always takes place in a pit somewhere—somewhere I never wanted to go with my patients and certainly nowhere I wanted to go for myself.

Yet on that first Sunday I was eager to make the voyage down. Whisked along in a wheelchair pushed by my Aunt Pat visiting from New York, I couldn't wait to meet the radiation therapist and subject myself to whatever ministerings he had planned for me.

The scene in the Radiation Therapy Department was very different from what I had imagined. The department office was bright and cheerful and the radiation therapist and his technician who awaited me were warm, personable, and reassuring. Feeling suddenly guilty for having dragged them in on a Sunday afternoon, I apologized for inconveniencing them. They dismissed my concern as they helped me out of the wheelchair. Their affability and light-heartedness as well as their command of a technology that could burn the tumor out of my chest made me feel immediately more hopeful. They had an elevator to transport stretchers and wheelchairs to the treatment level. I refused to use it, determined to walk the eight steps downward. With Aunt Pat steering me from behind, I made it.

Radiation meant the end of the line, and part of me expected the treatment room to be a dungeon complete with cobwebs on the ceiling, and chains to hold the patient in place. Again, the scene couldn't have been more different. The room, although clearly lined with lead and concrete, was large and comfortable. The floors were carpeted, the walls hung with thoughtfully selected paintings, and Muzak played in the background. In the middle of the room stood a sleek machine built like a massive upright question mark with a horizontal stretcher placed through its center. I climbed gingerly onto the stretcher and with the aid of several pillows arranged myself to receive the atomic potion. The therapists painted four indelible red marks on my chest indicating the boundaries of the radiation port, a twentieth-century scarlet letter, I thought. They left the room, bolting the heavy door behind them. Momentarily, they began talking to me on an intercom and assured me that I was not alone since they were watching me on a TV monitor. The therapy, they explained, would begin shortly, last for two and a half minutes, and be without sensation. I relaxed on the table as well as I could despite my various pains and swellings. I was happy that the hated malignancy was about to receive a counterattack.

Above me, originating from the bowels of the machine, I heard a faint sound like a small wave lapping on a beach. I fantasized that it was coming from a microscopic trapdoor opening that would let a tiny stream of radiation pass through. It was the only noise to be heard, and it soon stopped. There were no flashing lights, no revving motors, no futuristic fireworks. The colossal power of the machine set against its staggering silence seemed incredible to me. The things I thought of as powerful—bombs, trucks, engines, people—made noise, but this purveyor of cobalt-generated gamma rays was absolutely silent as it went about its chore. I felt nothing except for a faint warmth in my chest, which—like some distant light at night—disappeared when I focused hard on it. At the end of two and a half minutes the soft wave-lapping sound repeated itself and the treatment was over. The hydraulic doors opened, and Aunt Pat and the radiation therapist appeared to return me to the world of human beings once again.

The treatment continued every morning, five days a week, for six weeks. Although a non-physician technician took charge of the sessions, the therapist frequently showed up to visit with me. His attitude was invariably warm and thoughtful. At one point I asked him about this, since he was so different from my fantasy of radiation therapists. He responded that since he was generally dealing with such a frightening array of diseases, he felt that he had to work twice as hard as the average physician to support his patients. Moreover, since he was offering them a therapy that would likely extend or save their lives, he had reason to be optimistic and upbeat when working with them. He truly considered this his mission as a physician. His approach worked for me. His cheery, personalized attitude reinforced my belief in my own durability and prevented me from feeling like a marked person.

For Judy, too, the advent of my cancer meant drastic adjustments. Judy had been trained as a social worker and had been happily employed half-time at a child development center in Santa Fe. She devoted the balance of her efforts to caring for three-year-old Meghan. She too had grown to love the cross-cultural mountain beauty of northern New Mexico and thought of it as home. The illness was to change all that. Her career was revoked, her responsibilities as a parent were doubled, and the entire burden of family, financial, and household management fell on her. She became a harried diplomat working in the awkward middle-land between hospital, family, and outside world.

Much of this occurred without particular sympathy or support focused on Judy. She was not the *malade* but, rather, the heritor of all the disease's fallout—emotional, familial, and custodial. She was often treated as an also-ran in the tumor sweepstakes. I was to be the center of attention, the recipient of cards, messages, calls, and letters from friends, the specific object of people's concern. Judy's lot was to hold our lives together quietly and stoically. It was an awkward, difficult, and unsung task. She managed it beautifully.

I saw Meghan for the first time a week following the operation, about the time the swelling set in. A corpsman wheeled me down the long main corridor of the hospital to the first-floor lounge where she and Judy were waiting. She came running forward to me with a big smile on her freckled face. I could not get out of my wheelchair to greet her. I had an intravenous running in one arm and my coughing pillow was pressed to my heavily bandaged chest. The best I could do was reach out one hand to embrace her neck. "Hi, Daddy," she said. I began to cry. I tried to speak but I could not get out more than one or two words without a sob.

"Daddy, I brought you these." She handed me a fistful of crayon scrawls. She smiled again and I tried to thank her. Judy wheeled us into a corner of the waiting room where we could have a little privacy. The corpsman thoughtfully waited in the hallway where uniformed staff hurried one way and another.

"Meghan, I love you and I will get home soon to be with you," I tried to tell her through my tears.

"Daddy, does your neck hurt?" She pointed to the bandages rising above my pajamas. "Is that your *yaya?*" *Yaya* is Spanish slang for any kiddy injury. Through my tears I managed to chuckle at her expression, as did Judy. From that time on our familial nickname for the horrendous events occurring in my chest was the "Yaya." Though I tried to keep my emotions in check for the rest of our brief visit, I did not do too well. My tears came from some deep sense of weakness and emasculation that I neither understood nor could control. I was aware of the feeling that it was wrong to be vulnerable in Meghan's presence. If anything I should be just the opposite—strong and stoic. These thoughts were not reasoned on my part, they were instinctual and quite clear. For her to see me sick, unable to walk, unable, in fact, to do anything but spurt out a few acrid tears would, I felt, do damage to her image of me.

Meghan, though, seemed to take the situation in stride. My tears did not startle her. She accepted my being in a wheelchair because she knew that I was ill. And, after all, I mused later on, I had spent hours listening to her cry over the years. Crying was a strong emotion that we often experienced together. Nonetheless, I returned to my room resolved to control my emotions better at the time of our next visit.

In the weeks that followed I was to weep frequently and suddenly without immediate cause. The disease and its treatment so stripped me of my defenses that any event with the least bit of emotional content caused me to cry. I cried over some television news stories (Vietnam was falling at the time) as well as many kind letters that I received from friends. Talking with Judy about our future was always interrupted by a tearful episode or two on my part. While the tears were honest and cathartic they were also an annoying impediment to almost any serious conversation. In retrospect I suppose they were tears of impotence and anger, tears of a spirit that had been blindsided by disease. As the weeks passed, my raw emotions became rawer and my sense of self-pity deepened.

Generally, the physicians were straightforward in dealing with me. They called cancer cancer and openly discussed risk factors, side effects, and statistical probabilities, for which I am very grateful. The full extent of the damage to my chest was not presented as clearly as it might have been—a circumstance that would trouble me later—but the cancer itself was treated with salutary candor. I always had a good idea of what was happening and what to expect. I never felt circumvented or, worse, lied to. I could talk honestly with Judy or Mom and Dad with the full sense that everybody had the same information. We didn't have to waste precious energy protecting each other—them from me "finding out" and me from them suspecting that I "knew." I think this is far and away the best approach to serious illness but one that is often not followed. How much better to be able to speak candidly than to have to tiptoe awkwardly through the facts *and* the emotions at a time when family and friends can be terribly valuable in coping with a very tough reality.

The chemotherapy started three weeks following surgery. The chemotherapist, a judicious, balding oncologist, sat with me and discussed the possible drug treatments in somber tones. I appreciated his honesty and the forthright way he included me in the therapeutic discussions. His message was clear and simple. Seminomas can be cured, but the pathology of mine was "anaplastic," meaning that it was more dangerous and less predictable. Therefore, he suggested that the strongest drugs be used in a rigorous regimen. I consented, suffering a shudder of fear at the term "anaplastic," a word I had used casually enough before but which now had a particularly morbid personal meaning.

The medications were administered weekly in early-afternoon intravenous binges. The chemotherapist would select a vein, puncture it to draw off blood samples, and then inject in quick succession the three agents. The large quantities of clear, room-temperature fluid pouring into my arm produced a chilly sensation running up to my armpit. I wondered what my heart would do when the stream of blood to be recycled suddenly arrived severely diluted and contaminated with this cocktail of caustic chemicals. The heart never seemed to notice.

But the rest of the body did. Half an hour after the first dose, about the time I was arriving back in my room, I suddenly felt as if I had, indeed, been poisoned. I was overtaken by a malignant, pervasive sense of malaise, my temperature shot to 104° and remained there for several hours. Finally, I began to shiver violently, and slowly the temperature fell to normal. I was left colossally weakened, and by the next morning nausea and vomiting had set in, lasting for two or three days. The weakness remained throughout and was reinforced a week later by the next treatment, which produced similar results.

Chemotherapy was a paradox. The drugs were designed to kill tissue. Cancerous cells, which grow faster than most normal cells, tend to be more susceptible to these drugs. Nevertheless, they were poisons and behaved as poisons in the body. I hated them and yet at the same time they were one of the two lifelines that had been thrown me. Therefore I loved them. That irony was not lost on me as each week I felt the cold tingle running up my arm.

Generally I didn't carry on as doctors sometimes do when they become patients. I didn't bully the nurses, try to rewrite my orders, or challenge my medications. I had the opportunity to utilize manual skills of doctoring, though, from time to time in odd ways. When the multiple venipunctures that I received for IV's, blood specimens, and medications quickly exhausted my supply of large, easily entered veins, problems developed. The nurses soon became frustrated—as did I—with the difficulty (and pain) of starting IV's on me. I was a pediatrician by training and had started IV's in unbelievably small veins on the hands, feet, and scalps of infants. I figured that slipping a needle into my own vein wouldn't hurt any more than subjecting myself to someone else's often futile attempt. Junkies didn't seem to have any trouble. I wasn't wrong, and little by little, I became my own venipuncturist. I kept an eye on my IV fluids as well, and was not above adjusting the rates of flow when they were ahead or behind.

The Siege

The Naval Hospital has a movie theater, and one evening while I was still relatively strong, Mom was allowed to push me there in a wheelchair to see *The Towering Inferno*. I had a unit of blood running at the time, hanging from a pole attached to the wheelchair. Things went well for a while, but then the blood flow from the bag through my IV started to slow. One by one, I tried every trick I knew. I opened the line up wide. I changed the position of my arm and wiggled the needle this way and that. I coiled the IV tubing and squeezed it rhythmically in an effort to flush out any clots. Finally, I raised the support pole as high as possible to enlist the aid of gravity. Nothing worked. We had to give up and retreat to Tower Nine to enlist the help of a nurse just as the hotel in the movie was going up in flames.

As my treatments progressed, the subtleties of the doctor-turned-patient experience ceased to entertain me. The early fascination faded as I entered into what was indisputably a prolonged battle for my life, a battle in which my role seemed to be confined to bearing up under siege. My life consisted of fear, pain, and nausea in approximately equal parts and I withdrew further into my lachrymose shell. It is not with any pride that I portray myself during this period. I have thought a good deal about it since and wondered why I wasn't braver or more optimistic in my attitude. I have read about Hubert Humphrey padding around Memorial Hospital in New York with a belly full of tumor wishing good cheer to his fellow patients. I have read Norman Cousins writing persuasively about his own brush with terminal illness which he feels was cured in large part by laughter and vitamin C—both self-administered. Dr. Mills himself, at a later date, would gently chide me that had my attitude been more optimistic I might have healed more easily.

I only know that during this time I felt blighted physically and overrun psychologically. I am sure that deep within me I was furious at the fates which had brought me to my knees in youth. Had I had the energy and a target, or even a surrogate target, I imagine I would have broken out in rage. But I was past being angry. What I do remember feeling was despair. My glass, it seemed to me now, was indeed half empty. Why had I been singled out to receive this blow? Why would I not be able to see my grand-children or realize my full skills as a physician? Why would my parents have to see me, their eldest son, slowly die? Why did I have to vomit and tremble? Why was my hair beginning to come out by the combful? Why? Why?

A persistent question that I spent many restless hours mulling was the explanation for my cancer. There must be a reason—some comprehensible cause —I kept telling myself. I didn't just get sick. It seemed too unlikely. The disease had to be the logi-cal outcome of something—but what? I think I felt that the impact of the cancer would be lessened or made more bearable if I could find a rationale for it.

At times I entertained some fairly outlandish

thoughts. Just two weeks before my tumor was discovered, a friend had sent me a chain letter with a complicated set of instructions that included a brazen threat to the health of anyone who failed to send the letter on. People who had broken the chain, the letter warned, had experienced incredible misfortune in their lives. The letter even described some of these gruesome events. Early in my first hospitalization I suddenly remembered this letter and its grim message. I had not sent the letter on because I found its premise silly and its threat objectionable. Yet, later, casting about as I was for explanations, the letter assumed a new importance. Was I a victim of the supernatural—some malevolent and vindictive force disseminated by chain letter? This rationale never made sense to me but, in desperation, I spent a good deal of time wondering about it.

Guilt, also, was a theme in the search for a reason for my cancer. My plummet from youth and health to the depths of cancer must have been caused by something I had done . . . what was it? What act of hubris had I been guilty of? What principle, what ethic had I offended by my behavior? What had I done wrong? I never found sense or solace in these thoughts but I did entertain them. I mention them only to suggest that for me, as perhaps for others, the search for guilt is a natural and almost instinctive reaction to unforeseen disaster.

Several friends proposed another explanation for my illness: stress. More tangible than guilt but still a long way from anything like the germ theory of illness, stress was certainly much a part of my life before and, perforce, during my sickness. But cancer doesn't spring up like canker sores or pimples in students during exam week or diarrhea in soldiers in the trenches. Countless other young physicians experienced the pressures I did without becoming sick. I am persuaded that stress is a negative and complicating factor in our lives and one that deserves attention and redress, but it does not provide a simple explanation for my disease.

The scientific theory as to the pathogenesis of seminoma in the chest is still in the realm of speculation. It is known that early in embryonic life the cells that are destined to become gonadal tissue lie close to those that will develop into lungs. As the embryo grows, the gonadal cells—the so-called germinal ridge—migrate toward the pelvic area of the fetus and eventually differentiate into male or female sexual organs. The theory of mediastinal seminoma is that a number of cells are left behind in what becomes the chest of the fetus. These abnormally placed cells lie dormant for many years and then during adulthood become cancerous and begin to multiply rapidly.

I like the medical explanation of the seminoma since it absolves me of complicity in its origin and suggests that factors totally beyond my control determined its presence. Neither wrong doing nor wrong living has any place in a construct which blames the problem on the chance misplacement of a few cells in a microscopic ball of tissue more than thirty years ago.

If the disease wasn't my fault, then whose fault was it? My parents'? After all, they were responsible for my procreation and, according to the embryo-genetic theory the problem originated there. While my rational mind knows that errant cells within a fetus are not within the parents' control and by no measure are their "fault," it did give me a sense of relief to think, however irrationally, that the blunder belonged to someone else.

At one point when I was at my sickest and most desperate, I developed a vivid and urgent fantasy about returning to the womb. The problem lay there, I told myself, and the only true solution rested in returning to the site of the crime and starting all over again. Chemotherapy and radiation were after the fact and relatively useless. I felt like Humpty Dumpty with all the king's horses and all the king's men trying to mend me.

As I lay in bed struggling against nausea, my eyes wandering aimlessly over the input and output charts taped to the walls amidst Meghan's crayon sketches, I imagined starting all over again. It seemed so logical and so hopeful. This has all been a terrible mistake and it's ending so absurdly that we must simply stop and begin again. How, I wondered, would I get back inside? I was so damned big—so embarrassingly huge. And would Mom really want to go through it all again? She would have to participate. I knew I couldn't do it alone. Would she be willing to put up with another labor and delivery and a toddler and school and measles and all that over again? I felt she could be persuaded if she understood why, but the size problem was a real one. How would I ever get back inside? For days, through my worst bouts of nausea and depression, unable to eat and scared beyond reason, with Mom present and not present, I was obsessed with my return to the womb. This fantasy, wild as it was, helped me through some awful times. When all my rationality as a physician, as a patient, as a son told me that I was cornered, it gave me a way out. Gradually, as the worst effects of the therapy wore off and as the possibility of life reemerged, the fantasy became less frequent and less compelling.

The staff on Tower Nine stuck with me throughout as well as they could. Dr. Mills was persistently optimistic even though his surgical ministerings were a minor part of my care at this point. I grew close to some of the nurses and corpsmen who took care of me day in and day out. They coaxed me to eat and kept up my spirits and they counseled and encouraged my family. Some among the medical and nursing staff, however, were extremely curt with me, avoiding any kind of relationship. At first I assumed they simply disliked me. Eventually I talked to my friends on the staff about it and they explained that my presence on Tower Nine was difficult to handle since I was a peer in age and profession. Everyone was a bit self-conscious when dealing with me. My disease could easily have been their disease. I was no eighty-year-old retired sailor with lung cancer. I was one of them and I was sick as hell. Those members of the staff who could cope with this treated me evenhandedly and sympathetically. Those who could not tended to avoid me or bend over backwards to show indifference to my circumstances and discomfort. This simply fueled my sense of injustice and impotence at the time.

My feelings toward all the doctors involved in my care were, in fact, tinged with ambivalence. I was at once entirely dependent on them to save my life and angry with them for the errant biopsy that had come close to killing me. I wondered about the actual scene at the operating table when things went awry. Who was present at the moment and who actually wielded the biopsy forceps when the fateful bite was taken? Who did what next? Who were the heroes and who were the goats? I never asked these questions in any but a general way and I never received anything other than general answers. Yet, at the time, posing these questions bluntly to Dr. Mills or his staff would have seemed like an affront—an ungrateful challenge to the same people who were keeping me alive. Likewise, the notion of malpractice—the possibility that I would formally contest the performance of the surgeons—passed through my mind and out quickly because it seemed absurdly unappreciative of the salvage job they had done. These were dangerous, troubling thoughts for me, ones that threatened the tight, albeit tenuous, grip I had on life. For the time being I put them out of my mind but they were to return at intervals. A complete, graphic account of the surgery and its complications at some point during my treatment would have helped me deal with the surgical outcome and could have cleared up some of the divided feelings I had about the care I received.

I was feeling lonely and isolated. I had no friends or peers who were severely ill or who had cancer. I knew, of course, that cancers occurred in young adults but I knew of no one who was ill at the time. A close friend in grade school had died of leukemia, but that experience seemed hopelessly distant to me. Everyone else I knew was proceeding with his life and career. In my mind I was the only one who had been struck down with the kind of mortal illness that I associated with the elderly. I reflected bitterly that in my career as a physician my own diagnosis was, perhaps, the most tragic I ever made.

It is not true, of course, that only the elderly get cancer. There are a variety of cancers and other serious illnesses that afflict people in their twenties and thirties—seminoma among them. My particular sense of isolation, however, was reinforced by life on Tower Nine, where most of the patients were older military personnel who were undergoing cardiac bypass operations. Women were in the minority, young people were rare, and with one exception during that hospitalization, no one else had cancer. That one exception, significantly, became a close friend.

Commander Zwicker was a sixty-five-year-old retired naval officer. I got to know him because we both went to radiation therapy daily, and since he could walk and I could not, the nurses enlisted him as my "pusher." Each morning at 7:30 Zwicker would take command and navigate my wheelchair through the basement corridors of the Naval Medical Center with all the skill of his rank. My job was to carry our cargo, two large metal charts, on my lap. Our friendship grew around these trips but our bond was much deeper than that. It was our common disease.

Zwicker was a handsome man, lean, a touch gaunt, and always dressed in a paisley bathrobe which fit him well. He had been a merchant seaman once, captain of a vessel carrying cargo in the Caribbean. It had not been a very glamorous job, but it supported him and he did it well. At the outbreak of World War II his ship was commandeered by the Navy and he was given naval rank and naval authority. From that point on he became captain of a convoy vessel carrying military wares across the Pacific. The hazards were great. He had been fired on and torpedoed frequently. Nonetheless, he had come through it and stayed in the Navy for a career that concluded with a job at the Pentagon some five years before. He had retired and moved to Florida, where he was living happily and resourcefully until he encountered difficulty swallowing and was diagnosed as having a carcinoma of the esophagus. Like me, he had journeyed to Bethesda in search of the best the Navy had to offer. He was married and had children and grandchildren all around the United States. "Death," he told me, "is something I have faced several times. It is something that seeks you out or does not. There is really very little you can do about it most of the time. My attitude is to be as tough and as ordinary as possible in the face of it."

And tough and ordinary he was. The radiation bothered him not at all. He ate, walked, took daily passes from the hospital, and behaved in general as if nothing unusual was being done to him. We were quite frank talking to each other about our cancers. He consoled me with the fact that at my age as a naval captain he had faced death and that he was still around at this point and I very likely would be too. What attracted me to him most was not any formal bravado in the face of illness but quite simply his good spirits, which were always with him. He happily wheeled me through the hospital to our treatments, chitchatting about this and that, and then happily waited for me and wheeled me back. On Tower Nine he was always ready to talk, exploring any topic I wanted. He was, by his own definition, an ice-cream junkie, stashing away quantities of various flavors at all hours of the day and night. After his course of radiation he underwent surgery in an effort to remove as much of his esophageal tumor as possible. He tolerated the procedure splendidly and within several days he was up walking the halls again. Within a week he had his swagger back and was downing ice cream at a rapid rate. His spirit was always strong. He never seemed cowed by the maybes, the coulds, or the what ifs of his disease. He faced it head on and gamely.

Still, there was a major difference between Zwicker's situation and mine. He was sixty-five years old, a grandparent, and in retirement. His mission in life, I reflected, had been achieved, whereas mine, I was acutely aware, had not been. "Are you ready to die?" I asked him one day over ice cream. "I don't think anyone is ever *ready* to die," he responded. "I guess I'm ready to take what comes, but that doesn't mean I like what's happening."

I then tried out my ideas on him about how lucky he was to have finished his career and seen his family grow up. Suddenly, having grandchildren became the most important thing in the world to me. Zwicker chuckled. "Certainly I feel good about those things, but you're never done. I don't think most people are ever satisfied that they have accomplished everything they want to. To you sixty-five looks old. To me eighty looks old. To the eighty-year-old, ninety probably looks old. I'm not any more eager to be robbed of the next fifteen years than you are to lose the next thirty."

We were sitting in the "galley" on Tower Nine. He ate some more ice cream and I fingered a salt shaker on the Formica table. What he said was true but it did not remove the sense of embezzlement that was so much a part of my reality. I was glad for having done the things I had done, for having a daughter who would have some memories of her father, a wife to whom I had given some pleasure, and parents to whom I had given some pride. I had practiced medicine for six years and had, I hoped, given benefit to a number of patients. I had written the draft of a book that, with luck, would find its way into print. That was my tally sheet and in stoic moments I was happy with it. Zwicker's message was that the answer doesn't lie in tally sheets. Bench marks of achievement are much less the answer than are the simple satisfactions that come along with life. Counting his battle stars or polishing his medals while traveling in U-boat infested waters would have done him little good—then or now. Rather, life should be embraced resolutely in spite of the torpedoes, reaping such pleasure as friendship and good ice cream provide.

Zwicker left the hospital before I did to return to his home in Florida. He told me he looked forward to long walks on the beach. I have not heard from him since then.

I had never been a very religious person in any formal sense. Although raised a Catholic, I had not been active in the church for fifteen years. Judy and I had been married by a Unitarian minister and had cast about a bit in Santa Fe for a denomination that would be meaningful to us. When I had signed into the Naval Hospital, the registration card called for religious preference. I left it blank. As my illness progressed I wondered if my attitude about God and religion would change. Would I, faced with the prospect of death, find a piety or belief that had not been apparent in health? That did not happen. I grappled with my fate without benefit or burden of religious belief. It is hard to know whether that is good or bad, but it was natural for me. I think that while my experience with illness has made me more spiritual—teaching me, as it has, greater respect for the richness as well as the frailty of life—it has not made me more religious. To me the struggle was one of the human spirit and the human body. A formal God or formal religion simply did not play an important role in the events as I experienced them.

That is not to say that I did not receive attention or benefit from various clergymen. The Protestant chaplain, Rob Hill, who became involved with me and my family on the day of surgery, served as both messenger and counselor. He went on to become a good friend and frequent visitor throughout my illness. My parents, abiding by my Catholic roots, saw to it that I received the last rites in the operating room. Subsequently, the Catholic chaplain made my bed a way station on his daily rounds. A bald, friendly, awkward Navy captain, he gently tested my beliefs on his first visit. I assured him that I was not a practicing Catholic and that I did not plan to activate my religion for fear of dying. He said he respected that but asked if I would mind if he visited me anyway. I said I would not, and so he regularly

appeared at my bedside though we found little to talk
about. After several visits featuring many "How are
you's?" "OK's," and "God bless you's," he discovered
I was a stamp collector. It turned out that his hours
not spent in saving souls were devoted to philately
and this gave us a small plot of common ground
which he worked methodically. I remember few of
the details of our discussions except that his stamp-
collecting specialty was the Vatican. He was shopping for a parish in which to work when he retired
from the Navy, which was scheduled to happen
soon. His mixture of the secular (stamps, retirement,
and parish shopping) with the religious amused me,
although I'm afraid I was not a very satisfying subject for him.

One day a corpsman came into my room to tell me
there was a Reverend Smith to see me. I didn't know
any Reverend Smith and I wasn't feeling like company, but since he was standing at the nursing station on Tower Nine I felt that I could not say no.
Young, bearded, and wearing a black turtleneck jer-
sey, Reverend Smith arrived by my bedside. Around
his neck a wooden cross hung from a leather thong.
Reverend Smith was a born-again Christian dispatched by a friend of mine who had recently found
Jesus and could not resist the possibility that I might
too. Although Reverend Smith was gentle enough, I
recognized his style from the start. Like any good
salesman, he had a briefcase with literature that he
was eager to foist on me. He had a few precious
minutes to present his product. He worked quickly

and craftily to leave behind as many persuasive points as possible. On one level, I was deeply appreciative of his efforts and of the sense of caring that had motivated my friend to send him. On a more tangible level, however, I was uninterested in their product and peeved at the presumptuousness that would motivate them to proselytize me. In short, I was in no mood to be born again. I thanked the Reverend Smith for his attention and sent him and his wooden cross packing.

As my therapy continued through the spring, my condition became worse. The nausea was with me at all times and eating became a severe chore. To make matters worse, four weeks postoperatively I began to develop pain on swallowing. Very soon I became unable to swallow anything without severe pain. Liquid or solid, bland or not, any substance passing through my foodpipe caused acute pain. Water burned, antacids rasped, solid food stabbed. I could not even swallow my saliva—an annoying and humiliating situation. This state of affairs, subsequently diagnosed as a radiation burn of the esophagus, did little to support my physical or my mental well-being. I was reduced to eating baby food with the assistance of an oral anesthetic, an unctuous, foul liquid usually used for treating canker sores, which I would swallow by the teaspoonful, leaving my mouth feeling like cotton but enabling me to pass several spoonfuls of food into my nauseated stomach before the pain returned. I converted a green plastic hospital kidney basin into a spittoon, carrying it everywhere with me.

Sleep became almost an impossibility. My hourly catnaps were interrupted by bouts of vomiting and soaked pillows from feverish sweats and salivary overflow. My weight dropped off rapidly and I began to dread my twice-weekly trip to the scales. After six weeks of treatment, when I was losing weight at the rate of one pound a day and had lost a total of 35 pounds from my preoperative weight of 175, the oncologist decided to reduce my chemotherapeutic dosages and, soon after, to terminate them. A week later the total prescribed dose of radiation therapy had been achieved and it, too, was discontinued. The medical center had done what it could for me—surgery, radiation, and chemotherapy. The rest was up to my body and the fates. It was time to go home.

It was mid-May. Snow had all melted in the Sangre de Cristo Mountains in New Mexico. The cherry blossoms had bloomed and gone along the banks of the Potomac. Saigon had fallen. The tomato seeds I had carefully planted in cutaway milk containers in our kitchen in February were more than ready to be put in the ground. And La Clínica de la Gente had begun to look in earnest for a physician to take my place.

Judy had been busy during my hospitalization. Dr. Mills had counseled her that whatever the results of the therapy, there would be a period of continued treatment and observation. This would need to be done near a major medical center, preferably Bethesda. So Judy had bravely struck out on her own, found a house for rent in nearby Rockville, Maryland, returned to Santa Fe, loaded all our belongings into a moving van, rented our Santa Fe house, and returned East. With the help of her parents and mine she had moved into our new "home" in Rockville. Now she prepared to take her invalid husband there, yet another new experience.

Friends in the hospital congratulated me on my impending departure. I had made it through therapy and, after two months, was going home, where things would be better. I didn't feel that way about it at all. I had arrived at the hospital seemingly healthy, mentally intact, and ready to do battle. Now I was leaving the hospital in a wheelchair, emaciated, unable to swallow, troubled by breathing, and acutely depressed. I didn't miss my trips to the chemotherapy unit, but my last morning of radiation therapy, the day before I was to leave the hospital, I suffered an incredible spasm of anxiety. Crying did no good. Vomiting, spitting, and belching were in no way cathartic. There seemed to be no avenue of escape from the constant fear and nausea that I felt.

I began studying the screens on the two windows in my private ninth-floor room. Would I have the strength to remove them? Was there anything that I could lift that was heavy enough to punch through them? I didn't care so much where I landed or who discovered that I was missing as I did what the mechanism would be to get the windows cleared. I still had enough sense of what was going on inside my head to call the nursing station and ask for help. It was seven in the morning. Judy would be busy with Meghan, so I called Dad and asked him to come to the hospital as soon as he could. He was there by eight o'clock. In the meantime, a corpsman named Al who had been a steady friend sat beside my bed and held my hand. I hugged Dad when he arrived.

I had no idea of what was happening that day except that my life, or what was left of it, was coming to a head. In spite of my abhorrence of the hospital, I feared leaving it. The burning radiation and the noxious chemicals were what I had come to believe in—in spite of their poisonous effects. Deep within me I could not accept being cut adrift to fend for myself. I had become a slave of my therapies. Even though I understood the need to terminate them, I think I would have doggedly climbed onto the radiation table daily until the rays had burned a hole clean through me. Leaving Tower Nine through the window became more appealing than abandoning the poisons. I wanted to live at any cost, so badly, in fact, that I was prepared to die.

Going "home" seemed a hollow promise too. Where I was headed wasn't home, but a rented house in an unfamiliar neighborhood in a strange town. In no way was it like reclaiming my old life. It wasn't having a barbecue on Santa Fe Avenue or watching La Clínica's basketball team or visiting the familiar St. Vincent's Hospital in Santa Fe. I felt like I was leaving the hospital to go to some motel decorated with our furniture.

Until that day before my departure I had avoided psychiatric assistance in much the way I had declined the various religious offerings. But in my agitated state that morning I knew I needed help of some sort and I eagerly welcomed a khaki-clad Navy psychiatrist sent over as a consultant. He listened to my litany of troubles and then—without preamble—asked me if I would like to be held. I said yes. We sat together quietly for a few minutes clasped in an embrace, his hand patting my bony back. He smelled of after-shave lotion and his body was reassuring. My native embarrassment at being held by a man was totally overcome by my desperation. His sense of succor was so spontaneous, generous, and accurate that it still astounds me. Surely it came from no textbook of psychiatry but from the man himself.

Over the next three months I saw this doctor periodically in an effort to cope with my life as it continued. His counsel and his support were always valuable but never so crucial as that suicidal morning.

There were no mirrors in my hospital room, and while I knew I was losing weight, I had had no opportunity to see my body. Daily, to be sure, I showered and ran my hands over the increasingly bony prominences of myself, but somehow that didn't add up to what had really happened until I came home and saw myself in a full-length mirror. I was staggered. My arms, once strong, stuck into the sides of my chest like broomsticks on a scarecrow. My buttocks had turned soft and fleshless and my leg muscles— the legs I had once been proud of—had been replaced by loose hanging flesh. My waist was terribly concave, sucked in over the immutable hip bones. I ran my hands over my body with a new appreciation of what Judy had been watching. I had *felt* sick. Now I saw what it was like to *look* sick.

The problems created by my condition were more than cosmetic. First of all, I had trouble sitting on anything hard. The flesh on my buttocks had been so reduced that a wooden chair or a park bench was terribly painful to sit on—and that is no small problem for someone as dependent on sitting as I was. Walking the distance of half a block tired me to the point that I had to sit down; stooping to pick up a sock was a chore to be contemplated, planned, and then executed delicately. Getting off the toilet could be taxing.

Sometime after leaving the hospital I was standing in front of our new house watching a large bully of a neighborhood cat chase Brooklyn, our elderly, eccentric pussy. As I bent down to pick up an empty beer can that had been left on the street, and threw it at the marauding feline, I thought my entire arm would come off. I was in pain, the can went no more than six feet, and the cat escaped unscathed.

I lived in a new body, a body produced by cancer

and cancer treatment. My new condition called for an adjustment I could never have imagined. Judy patiently nursed me through this terrible time, heating the baby food, fixing milk shakes, keeping Meghan diverted so I could sleep, encouraging me to walk that half block I could manage in front of the house, and taking me on drives to nowhere in particular. Judy's parents, Dorothy and John Wentworth, spent much of the early months of my illness in Washington helping Judy and Meghan with the various rearrangements that had to be made. John had returned to Minneapolis before I left the hospital, but Dorothy stayed on into the summer, joining us in our new house. Supportive in every way, she helped run the household, freeing Judy to spend more time with me. She also proved to be a crafty weight-watcher, putting her cunning to work by slipping unsuspected eggs into my milk shakes and presenting me with bowls of ice cream or glasses of high-protein supplement when I least expected them. My sister Quita took me for car rides and indulged me with marvelous, lengthy, mind-numbing back rubs. When my brother Tony visited, he roughhoused with Meghan, giving her "airplane rides" and tickles, which she loved. Mom arrived daily, running endless errands and boosting spirits with interesting newspaper clippings or fresh vegetables for the house. Dad bought us a new color TV—our first!—and we watched the Washington Bullets—a team I had not yet learned to love—breeze through the national Basketball Association play-offs, only to be clobbered in the championship series by the Golden State Warriors. It was a team effort to keep me sane and begin to put the pounds back on.

But it was not to be an easy course. I was again receiving chemotherapy—a "maintenance" dose—every three weeks. My esophageal burn remained unchanged on into the summer. Although the nausea diminished and my appetite was starting to return, the discomfort and difficulty of eating prevented me from regaining any weight. With three "meals" a day and periodic forced snacks, I just barely maintained myself at 140 pounds, 35 pounds underweight. It was quite clear to everyone, including me, that if I could not start to put some flesh back on my very protuberant bones, I would not be able to recapture my strength. Unquestionably, food was my drug of choice.

A new problem began to emerge at this point: I began to be obsessed with the question of whether the tumor would reappear. This is a problem shared by all cancer patients. Unlike an infectious disease that can be eradicated by treatment with antibiotics, recurrence of cancer is always a real possibility. In fact, the fear of the disease can be as bad as the disease itself. I realized that it was possible, as Dr. Mills had encouraged me to think, that there was no living cancer in my body. I tried hard to focus on that, but I still felt like a child walking through a dark forest. In spite of reassurances that there are no goblins in the woods, the walk is still very frightening. Ultimately I knew that Dr. Mills couldn't be

sure whether there were goblins or not. And so, fear-
fully, humorlessly, I began to study my body, wondering where they might show up.

Not simply content to examine my scar from time
to time, I put my medical knowledge to work against
myself. I couldn't shave without finding a distended
blood vessel or sleep without suffering a "night
sweat." I attached a morbid diagnosis to every lump
or rash I could discover. In addition, I mentally performed an examination to go with each new "finding." I put myself through exploratory operations,
liver biopsies, and brain scans. Unable to seize on the
positive, I wallowed in the negative.

My spirit and my stamina were painfully low during the long summer of 1975. Recalling it now reminds me of how hobbled a potentially vital human
being can become under the assault of disease. The
experience has left me acutely aware of the special
apprehensions of cancer patients who are frequently
compromised in their ability to take gratification
from life—as I was. For them, the gnawing, self-
consumptive fear of recurrence is a constant and de-
structive phenomenon.

The particular loneliness of the cancer patient got
to Judy before it got to me. One Sunday she read a
newspaper article describing a cancer group, a number of cancer patients getting together to discuss
their illnesses. She thought it might be a good idea
for us. In fact, we both spent a good deal of time

engaged in brooding about my illness but relatively little time discussing it in a constructive fashion. We talked periodically with the doctors about my tests and symptoms. We answered the gentle questions of family and friends about my situation and prognosis on a regular basis, but much of that was repetitious and well defended for both their sake and ours. Quietly, each to ourself, we mulled the grim possibilities about the future but tended to avoid frank discussion with each other about some of our greatest fears.

I think we wanted to get those fears out and have an opportunity to compare notes with other people going through similar experiences. We weren't living in a retirement community where many families were dealing with serious or terminal illnesses. The various issues our friends were dealing with—children, divorce, careers—were serious, but they were not death and debility. In retrospect, a cancer group was just the thing for us, although at the time I was reluctant. I didn't particularly want to tell people about my illness and I was embarrassed by the spittoon that went everywhere with me. Moreover, I still clung to a certain medical chauvinism that said that I knew more about my disease than other patients would know about theirs. My altruistic and clinical instincts were in abeyance and I had little urge to help others cope with their diseases and little sense that they would be able to help me with mine. Finally, I suppose, I wasn't really wild about associating with "cancer patients." They had their problems and I had mine and I was reluctant to see them in any measure as the same.

Cancer groups are not common. It took Judy a good deal of research to locate one in the Washington area. The American Cancer Society sponsored no such activities at that time, but a helpful telephone receptionist had heard of a local cancer group and gave Judy a phone number. She called immediately and enrolled us. The group had been started a year or so earlier by Dr. Herb Manley. Thirty-five, bearded, and athletic, he was a practicing oncologist in the Washington area. All of the participants except for me were patients from his practice. His basic concept was that in the midst of his busy practice he did not have adequate time to explore, let alone support, the emotional needs of his cancer patients. Therefore, he set aside a two-hour evening period every two weeks and selected patients were invited to take part in a group discussion. Everyone was to bring a "loved one," usually a spouse, but brothers, sisters, and lovers were also present. We were a varied crew, young and old, apparently healthy and not so healthy, men and women, retired and child rearing. Manley, an amateur but warm and knowledgeable group leader, coordinated the sessions.

Mary (we used first names immediately and exclusively) was a woman in her fifties with a husband at least ten years her senior. She had had a mastectomy several years earlier and was suffering from recurrence of the cancer. Her left arm was grotesquely swollen and virtually unusable. That much was obvious. Additionally, she reported that the scar on her chest had broken down and was festering with malignancy. At each meeting she told of the very tangible progress of her illness. Her attitude was weary and resigned. Her husband seemed more depressed than she was, although it was difficult to tell since he talked little. Slowly they were losing the battle to maintain their lives intact. They had sent their teenage son to live with relatives because Mary felt she was not up to caring for him. Her husband was in retirement and did nothing but vaguely look after himself and assist with Mary's needs. "I mow the lawn," he answered in response to an inquiry as to what he did with his time. "When Mary feels too bad sometimes I do the dishes. We watch a lot of TV."

I was never able to tell Mary and her husband how sad their condition made me feel. I suppose, in a way, we all spend our time making do and waiting for the inevitable, but stripped of passion, shorn of activities, and pursued in a vacuum, life becomes horribly barren. Add to that a graphic, malignant clock ticking in the decaying skin of an ex-breast and that described Mary's life. I resolved that whatever happened to me I would never send my children away and die watching TV.

Buck was every bit as diseased as Mary but his life was quite different. He had the meaty wrists and forearms of an athlete, which indeed he had been. Fifty-five years old, a former professional hockey player, until recently he had had reason to anticipate a number of years of continued health and sportsmanship. During the past three years, however, he had been diagnosed as having not one, but two separate cancers—leukemia and cancer of the prostate. The side effects of his treatments did little to cool his ardor for the Baltimore Orioles, the Washington Bullets, or his golf game. He described with considerable insight and humor how his interests had continued to stimulate him in spite of his diagnoses. But athletic occupational therapy did not prove a simple solution for Buck. His golf game had been grounded following a heart attack on the golf course six months earlier. Undaunted, he had ignored medical advice and returned to the greens with the aid of a golf cart. Still the fates refused to cooperate with Buck. Recently he had developed a large and uncomfortable hernia. In view of his heart condition as well as the chemotherapy he was receiving, the surgeons declined to operate, so Buck was left with season tickets to the Orioles and the Bullets to satisfy his sporting needs.

Buck was very funny as he described his many medical problems, most of which were camouflaged by his robust appearance. "I can't get wrung out over cancer. I've got so many troubles the others would get jealous. One of them—or all of them—will get me sooner or later, so why worry about it? I've got better things to do with my time."

Anthony, the group's only black member, was a middle-aged ring maker. He never wore fewer than eight rings on his fingers, but counting the ones hung from his neck, he frequently arrived wearing twenty. Usually he came carrying a small, felt-lined box with more of his wares for show and sale. He exuded warmth and joviality and at first it seemed to me that he had no illness at all but came as some sort of artsy co-therapist. In time I learned that in fact he was extremely weak and was suffering from multiple myeloma—a cancer of the bone marrow. He carried his disease so easily that it seemed the group was more of a foil for his artistic talents than a support for his illness. "That's wrong, man," he countered when I told him my feelings. "That's just plain wrong. These rings *are* me. If you look at them, if you hold them, if you put them on your fingers, that's me. I'm not big at talking about a lot of this stuff but this group is where it's at for me. I make rings, sure. But I got cancer and you all understand about that. You're important to me. This is where it's at." I liked Anthony for his bluntness.

The group did have young members. There were four other people under forty, including two younger than I was. I was encouraged seeing this at my first session because the isolation that I had felt as a young person with cancer had been considerable. I looked forward to comparing my travails with these people in particular. All of them were women and, as it turned out, all of them had breast cancer and had undergone a mastectomy. Obviously this experience gave them a tremendous amount in common and really constituted them as a group within the larger group. This became quite clear when Gayle joined shortly after I did. Aged thirty-six, she was recovering from a radical mastectomy. Much of her first session was devoted to the other breast-cancer patients sharing their particular experiences with her. They offered her an educated discussion of the pros and cons of radiation therapy, advice on what to do with your children on the down days following chemotherapy, and shopping pointers on where to purchase breast prostheses. Gayle discovered a complete support system waiting for her that was something very special and different, I think, from what the rest of us with less specific tumors encountered when we arrived in the group.

I had real trouble with this because of my disappointment. Had I met any of these women outside of the group I think we would have found a tremendous amount in common because of our ages and our conditions. That intimacy was lessened for me within the group because the closeness among the women that was based on their disease and its social stigma left me at a distance. Breast cancer is, perhaps, a paradigm of a young person's cancer because it involves scarring, an assault on sexual identity, and problems with child rearing in addition to all of the other elements of cancer-patienthood. The women in the group who had undergone mastectomy welcomed newcomers into their circle warmly and deftly. My problem, as I discovered my resentment, was that I was facing those very same issues and sought the same helpfulness and clubbiness. Yet they didn't see me as one of their members for a number of understandable reasons. In spite of my youth and my chest scars and my young child, they saw my disease as being as distant from theirs as Mary's or Buck's or Anthony's.

My initial excitement at meeting these women was followed by a period of cynicism. Judy chided me for my callous attitude when I called them "the Breasties." Later on I began to understand the reason for my feelings and I accepted more easily their togetherness. My reaction, though, alerted me to the need I was feeling to share and compare my own experiences. I still saw most cancer patients as older folks. Commander Zwicker had been enormously helpful—but from the distance of a generation away. I wanted to ask someone—someone like me—how to get back to work feeling the way I did, what the kids would grow up remembering, how to kick the spittoon, what to do on a beach with a Terry-and-the-Pirates scar from Adam's apple to mid-back, and many more questions.

Among the mastectomy patients in the group there was a special person who stood out as a bit of a guru for all of us. Joan was a forty-five-year-old warrior who had undergone not one, but two mastectomies, two divorces, and lost her adrenals and ovaries in a twenty-year battle against breast cancer. Highly articulate and well informed, Joan had undergone virtually every permutation of breast cancer and its therapies and knowledgably shared these experiences with the group. She had tried standard drugs and experimental drugs, she had studied and dismissed Laetrile, she had been in psychotherapy and had practiced both Zen and Yoga. She had continued to work during much of her therapy but had recently been formally retired from her government job. In spite of all that, the disease still stalked her and in a dramatic revelation one evening she described to us how a recent lymph-node biopsy had proved malignant.

Dr. Manley deferred and referred to Joan frequently. She had had her first mastectomy, she pointed out gently, when the oncologist was still in high school. She used her knowledge and experience in a thoughtful and mature way, never talking down to other members of the group. She was the advocate, par excellence, of making every moment count. Since she had lived in the shadow of her disease for two decades, she was clear about the need to extract pleasure and meaning from life as one went on. "Can you imagine," she told the group one day, "what my life would have been like if I had deferred my happiness for a clean bill of health? I would have been in a twenty-year funk with no end in sight. If I have learned any lesson, it is: Don't wait for the doctor to make you happy. You're the only one who can do that, and often you have to do it in spite of what the tests are telling you."

That message didn't rest well with me at the time as I shifted uncomfortably on my fleshless buttocks trying to spit discreetly into my spittoon (I had converted to a small ceramic vase for social occasions). I still felt bitter about the simple good health that I was missing. My disease infuriated me. But Joan was right; although I had trouble digesting it then, my rage served me no useful purpose. Joan's basic point for cancer patients—or, for that matter, for everyone —is a simple and good one. Live the life you have left and don't wallow in memories or speculations about what life might have been or ought to be.

But positive attitudes could be counterfeit or at least suspect as well. Susan was a thirty-two-year-old mother of two with a graying high school teacher for a husband. She had undergone a mastectomy seven months earlier and now was certain that she was cured—something she tried to hammer home half a dozen times at each meeting. Susan had a solution for every problem discussed by the group and she was endlessly opinionated about cancer therapies. She had overcome depression, licked sadness, triumphed over fatalism, crushed anxiety . . . in short, had beaten her disease in every physical and emotional way possible. A session did not pass without Susan reassuring the group that mastectomy was no reason to doubt your sexual self. She would end by massaging her breasts to demonstrate to everybody that her new one was indistinguishable from the old.

Susan's husband tended toward silence. His demeanor was glum and I wondered if he did not bear the burden of anxiety for both of them—his recognized and hers denied. He never challenged her or her endless happily-ever-after babble, but I felt that underneath he was as angry at his wife's attitude as I was. The group was reluctant to challenge Susan's obsessive positiveness. Gingerly, one session, Dr. Manley asked her if she really believed all of the things she said. Then several others joined in a chorus that gradually became openly critical. A persistent complaint was articulated by one group member who said, "If you're so damned certain about everything why do you bother to come to the group? Why do you spend so much time talking? You take up a lot of my time and I'm *not* so sure about my future." Susan denied any motives other than a sense of well-being. She was quiet for the balance of that meeting, but in subsequent weeks her self-supporting garrulousness returned to its previous level. Even if the group did not change Susan's behavior, her presence was beneficial for the rest of us because watching her wrestle endlessly with her own fear, denying it in every way possible, taught us a lot about our own fears.

Dr. Manley was a benevolent mystery to me. Immersed as he was in oncology fifty to sixty hours a week, it was remarkable to me that he would choose to give still more of his time to the group. Indeed, he gave not only his time but his office space, as well as beer and coffee.

"Herb," I asked him once after a meeting, "why do you do this?"

"Do what?"

"Give your evenings over to cancer sessions after you have already spent all week talking to cancer patients."

"That's a definite problem I have," he responded.

"A busy oncologist doesn't spend much time *really* talking to patients. The pace of life at the office and the hospital is so quick that I rarely get the kind of time I want to talk to people about their troubles and how they are coping. That's the difference between an oncologist and almost any other kind of physician. The pace of any doctor's routine may rule out time for much intimate discussion with patients, but then the average condition in general practice is going to heal fairly easily anyway. Flu, diaper rash, ulcers, even the bottle . . . all of them warrant the talking but none of their treatments will suffer badly without it. The people I see are different. They all have a reason to fear for their lives. Their anxieties are rarely inappropriate or overdrawn. On the contrary, they're probably not dealing with their illness if they *don't* have some fairly basic questions about their lives. That's difficult for me because I would like to be able to talk about future plans and family troubles and all the rest—and not just the dose of chemo or the X-ray results."

Manley was dead right about that. The oncologist who cared for me spent little time on anything but the details of my treatment and disease. His waiting room was always packed and he always ran behind. I rarely felt that he had the time or the inclination to listen to what concerned me beyond the drug reactions or my weight fluctuations. His office was a place to receive medical treatment, not counseling or support.

"So this group at least lets me work closely with

certain of my patients. It teaches me, too. I have not yet had cancer." There was always a certain fatalism in his remarks when he talked about cancer and himself. "Listening to my patients, really listening to them, helps me to know more about what it is like. The group is making me a better doctor."

On the way down in the elevator after a meeting, one group member insisted that Dr. Manley had a fascination with death, which was the real reason he had become an oncologist and spent his energies on the group. Although that possibility did afford a simple explanation of the young doctor's commitment, I thought it was inaccurate. Certainly Manley had a tolerance for the severely ill or he would not have been a cancer specialist. But, beyond that, he was compassionate and concerned for his patients in an extraordinary way. Not satisfied with the standard limits of doctoring, he labored to help his patients cope with their diseases and live as fully as they could. Far from being a morbid preoccupation, Manley's practice was affirming of life. Judy and I attended the group for several months. It helped us to deal with the realities of cancer—realities we saw reflected in the perceptions and trials of the rest of the group.

As we were driving through the parking lot of a shopping center one day, the smells of a Chinese restaurant reached me and produced a pang of nostalgic hunger. Suddenly Chinese food became a dazzling goal for me. If only I could have the exquisite pleasure of once again eating Moo Shu Pork or Hot and Sour Soup, I would never forget—*never* forget what it had been like when I could not eat them. The frivolity, the license, the freedom of being able to eat Chinese food became a symbol of health recaptured for me.

Slowly, by the middle of summer, several months after the end of radiation, the discomfort from swallowing began to recede. One day we went to dinner at Mom and Dad's house and without consulting me they cooked a cube steak, cut it in tiny pieces, and presented it to me with a bowl of meat juice. It smelled wonderful and with them urging me on I managed to get most of it down. A delicious victory!

Soon after that, Judy and I spent a weekend at the shore visiting with our friends the Kindigs. Judy bought a dozen oysters and Dave Kindig hammered the shells open, since we didn't have a proper knife. Again, in spite of my balky foodpipe, the oysters looked tempting. I had not taken a bite of anything as big as an oyster in four months, but the prospect of cutting an oyster into bite-sized morsels seemed silly, so I resolved to tackle one whole, without either cocktail sauce or my anesthetic mouthwash. That oyster tasted different from any other oyster I have eaten, before or since. The average oyster is slurped, swallowed whole without benefit of chewing. At heart, I think most people are squeamish about oysters. I have been a slurper, I confess. But I chewed this oyster carefully and intently and it provided me with a complete marine experience. As I chewed I could taste salt marshes, sea breezes, the seaweed at low tide, salt spray, and the dunes. Both families watched as I took it on and, when I swallowed it, we all rejoiced.

Toward the end of the summer, the doctors encouraged me to get away from Washington for a while. The intervals between doses of chemotherapy were three weeks—enough time for a real trip. So we packed up the three of us and flew to New Hampshire to join Judy's parents at their cabin on the shore of Lake Sunapee. There we spent the time taking walks, fishing, and eating. Dorothy cooked wonderfully and coaxed me at every meal, so that, marvelously, a pound at a time, my weight started to climb. When we arrived back in Washington I had retrieved ten precious pounds and my strength and attitude reflected it. Shortly after our return we celebrated by going to a Chinese restaurant.

It was as delectable as I had hoped.

CHAPTER
3
___

Caitlin

The National Naval Medical Center is surrounded by a park-like campus with nicely planted court-yards and landscaped gardens. The area in front of the hospital is maintained as a golf course with a small pond in its midst circled by a walk. During that first spring while I was still a resident of Tower Nine, Mom and Judy would frequently coax me out of the hospital to sample a bit of the new season that was greening all around. They would wheel me to a courtyard for a brief stroll or sit me in the sun in my wheelchair.

Spring felt strange and alien. I recognized her sensuous breezes and playful sunlight but they did little to inspire my embattled body. I felt a bit cheated as I sat dumbly in my bathrobe or tottered a few paces in my slippers. Spring had always been a lusty time for me, lusty and ardent. But in the spring of 1975 I was a medical POW and I had no lust or ardor with which to greet the balmy Maryland May.

Four weeks into my hospitalization Judy announced that her period was two weeks overdue. My first response was as a clinician. Stress and worry are among the most frequent causes of delayed or absent menstruation. This was merely her body's way of showing concern for our situation, I reassured her. She would have her period soon. The possibility of pregnancy seemed remote and unthinkable.

Soon after that, in late April, Judy returned to New Mexico to arrange for shipment of our household goods East. She stopped in at La Clínica and had them run a pregnancy test on her. She called me that night and announced simply: "I *am* pregnant." The effect on me was staggering. I was at once joyful and overwhelmingly sad. I was delighted, as was Judy, that she had our baby inside of her, yet I found it unspeakably painful that I might well never see the birth of the child. It suddenly seemed to me that a quintessential human tragedy would be to sire an infant whom I would never see and who would never know me.

We congratulated one another on the phone and wondered aloud together what we should do. We agreed to postpone the discussion until she returned to Washington and we could talk face to face. When she arrived in my hospital room several days later, we clasped each other tearfully in one of our most intimate embraces ever. The decision we had before us was a momentous one, really a decision of life itself. She wheeled me down to an empty orthopedic clinic where we sat on the plastic chairs and mulled our situation. She sipped Coke out of a can and I spat into my kidney basin.

We could keep our secret, end the pregnancy, and remain as we were. Or we could let nature take its course both with the child and with me. On balance I felt good about the pregnancy. If I was to live, it was definitely something I wanted, and if I was to die, I felt I would like to leave the additional legacy of another child. The ultimate decision, though, was Judy's. She had to face the possibility of being a single parent, of having to explain death to a toddler, of sharing her precious reserves between Meghan and the unborn infant. Judy fingered her Coke and paced back and forth. Painfully, carefully, we explored every aspect of the situation. The phenomenon of the conception was astonishing to us then and remains so now since for almost a year Judy and I had wanted another child but, to our frustration and disappointment, nothing had happened. When we had come to Washington in the shadow of the newly discovered tumor, the thought of babies or birth control had never crossed our minds. We knew the immediate future looked bleak and the night before I entered the hospital we allowed our passion one final tryst. Unexpectedly, incredibly, beautifully, the seed took root.

I really never doubted the decision that Judy would make. Whatever the outcome of my cancer, whatever the risk, whatever the burden, she wanted the child and she was willing to raise it alone if necessary. It was a gutsy but predictable stance on Judy's part. Life would go on no matter what. We left the orthopedic waiting room eager to share our remarkable secret with the world.

We arranged to have Mom and Dad visit the hospital the next evening when Judy was there. A gentle spring rain fell outside Tower Nine and I had, as usual, sent my dinner tray back to the kitchen without having eaten much. We asked Mom and Dad to get chairs and sit by the bed, since we had something important to tell them. Nothing, I am sure, could have been further from their minds than the thought of pregnancy. They sat dutifully by the bedside of their gaunt son. They looked at Judy, hale and handsome in tidy slacks, long hair tied back in a ponytail. They looked at their son's hollow cheeks, bony shoulders, sallow skin, and waited for whatever news we could possibly have to tell them at this juncture in our lives. What was left?

"Judy is pregnant," I announced.

They were astonished and jubilant. All of us, really, were overwhelmed as we fell to congratulating and hugging one another. All four of us cried a bit in the deliriousness and surprise of the moment.

From the start, they took the news as total affirmation of life, not doubting our decision for a moment. The family was being extended and that was cause enough for celebration—indeed, the circumstances were reason for redoubled enthusiasm. Their elation confirmed our sentiment that life was triumphing over death. To all of us the pregnancy seemed to be a wonderful omen that invoked not only the powerful joy of the first awareness of a new life but, in our case, the renewal of an old one as well. When they went back out into the wet night we were all very happy—certainly happier than at any time since my surgery.

We called Judy's parents, who were back in Minnesota, and they, too, were delighted and supportive. The next morning I told Dr. Mills and the word traversed Tower Nine in less than an hour. For the next several days Judy and I were subjected to a steady stream of felicitations from fellow patients, doctors, nurses, and corpsmen. I felt as if I had won a Pulitzer Prize or a Medal of Honor. Among the most ebullient were the radiation tech who administered my daily treatment and the cleaning woman who dusted my room. Several doctors and nurses whom I knew only slightly or who had not previously been particularly friendly went out of their way to offer their best wishes. The idea of paternity for a cancer patient seemed to affect everyone who heard about it.

The baby gave a focus to my life that had been lacking. In spite of the pain, in spite of the spittoon, in spite of the nausea, I now knew that I must live until at least December of 1975 so that I could see our new child.

In the months following my discharge from the hospital, I wanted very much for Judy and me to be a team. Although severely limited in my capabilities, I was determined to be a good father and husband and to support Judy as much as possible through her pregnancy. In the early months, however, my resolve generally surpassed my abilities. Fortunately, Judy was strong and gamely added pregnancy to her other responsibilities. She ran the house, swam regularly, and took care of Meghan and me. As her pregnancy advanced it became more difficult for her to do many of the household chores. I would scold her for lugging groceries from the car up the back stairs into the kitchen because it was not good for the pregnancy. At the same time I had difficulty with heavy bundles myself and wasn't much help, my sense of gallantry far exceeding my capabilities. I agonized over the possibility of our car getting a flat tire, which I couldn't change and she shouldn't, but fortunately our tires held out during this critical passage. Meghan became more and more useful as chief stooper and bender and daily I would herd her around the house to pick up everything on the floor.

One night in July, well into the pregnancy, Judy woke me to say she had begun to bleed. We were both scared as we lay in bed and listened to the first morning birds and pondered the unthinkable—miscarriage. We said very little to each other, but there in the dark the same painful possibilities crossed our minds. The new baby meant something special to us—a symbol of life, a rugged commitment to carry on. In addition to what any pregnancy means, this one was a symbol and statement for both of us. All of a sudden we were faced with its loss. All that it had come to mean stood to be erased. The chirping birds were oblivious to our pain as the windows brightened and the day broke upon us.

Judy visited the obstetrician that morning. His prescription was bed rest, patience, and hope. I was simply not strong enough to manage the house, along with cooking and caring for Meghan, so various members of my family as well as several neighbors pitched in with cooking and child care. With their help we made it through an extremely difficult week. Slowly the bleeding stopped with no miscarriage. Little by little, Judy got back on her feet and we returned to our routine. The nameless, teasing fate that had toyed with us moved on.

That summer Judy took up swimming with a passion. She looked healthy, brown, and plump in her flowered bathing suit as she headed out across our lawn to the neighborhood pool. In one hand she lugged her bag of paraphernalia, in the other she carried Meghan's water wings. Meghan bobbed after her, babbling endlessly. In a bathing suit, Judy's growing belly was particularly obvious to the three-year-old and she asked about it. We explained to Meghan that Mommy was going to have a baby and that the baby was in Mommy's tummy. She immediately grasped the idea, explaining to us she was going to be a big sister. The idea appealed to her and she repeated it frequently in the following months.

Gingerly at first, but with increasing regularity, I too attempted mild forms of exercise. Twice a day I would walk the length of our block and back and periodically I would weed and prune in our vegetable garden in the back yard. Bending wasn't easy, but once I was situated on the ground I was as good a picker as I had ever been. Late in the summer I tried swimming. Since I had lost so much fat from my body, I found even the most tepid swimming-pool water to be frigid. Moreover, with the fat missing I found it extremely difficult to stay afloat and the energy required for swimming to be much greater than it had ever been before. The result was a great deal of chilly work for very little accomplishment.

In all these activities, walking, gardening, and swimming, I noticed that I became winded easily. For instance, walking to the end of my block at anything more than an amble left me breathing hard. Swimming half a dozen strokes not only caused me to breathe hard but in order to regain my wind I had to lift my chest out of the water. When I raised these problems with Dr. Mills he acknowledged that the radiation had destroyed a certain amount of the lung tissue in my central chest. Moreover, the extensive surgery and the subsequent internal scarring had diminished the capacity of both my lungs. Finally—and he showed me my X-ray to demonstrate it—my right diaphragm was paralyzed. In the effort to stop the bleeding and remove the tumor, my right phrenic nerve had been severed. "Under the circumstances, there was no way we could have avoided it," he explained. "It was just part of the surgery." I was stunned. The phrenic nerve has but a single purpose and that is to stimulate the bellows-like effect of the diaphragm, which, when contracting downward, sucks air into the lungs. Since my right phrenic nerve was gone, my right diaphragm had assumed a comfortable but useless position well above its normal location. The bellows was gone and my right lung was largely functionless.

These revelations certainly squared with the breathlessness I felt when doing anything the least bit athletic. My lungs angered me—or rather my lack of lung power angered me. I spent a good deal of time concentrating on the right side of my chest trying to imagine what was not happening within it. I fancied a warm, inert feeling beneath my right breast corresponding to, I thought, my limp lung. Whether the feeling was real or not, I spent a lot of mental energy chastising my chest for what it wouldn't do ever again. Some tissues in the body, when damaged, will regenerate. The liver and the intestine are good examples of bodily parts that have nine lives or more. Nerve tissue and lung tissue, as it happens, have but a single life. Once damaged they do not regenerate to any significant degree. I would have to make do with such breathing apparatus as I had left.

I was struck by the paradox of this one day toward the end of summer while lying down, gazing at Judy's swollen belly. I was thinking how much larger it looked than it had several weeks before. That meant, obviously enough, that the baby was growing, building new organs, and making new tissues. Suddenly it occurred to me that the baby, my offspring, my creation, was right at that moment developing lung buds and growing lung tissue itself. Deep within Judy's womb, a child of mine, a sperm of mine, cells of mine were reproducing and modeling themselves into tissues that I could not produce myself. My child, as yet unnamed and unknown, was doing something that I could not do and yet desperately needed done. It was a realization that made the generation gap as tangible as ever it would be. This would not be the last time that my child would do something that I could not do, but it certainly was the first and it struck me as a biological event of momentous proportions.

Judy and I were natural-childbirth buffs. We had read the books and taken the course in preparation for Meghan's birth. It had been a good experience and we wanted to do it again. So, in October, when Judy was six months pregnant, we enrolled in a Lamaze course to bring our technique up to snuff. It was good for us in many ways. With the exception of our evenings with the cancer group, it was the first time since my illness that we had ventured out regularly together as a couple. Every Tuesday night for six weeks we had a guaranteed date. The babysitter came, we threw pillows and blankets in the back of the car and headed off into the night like teenagers making for the drive-in. Our destination, however, was the linoleum floor of the library of a nearby grade school. There we were lectured and rehearsed by a Lamaze team, a tall, attractive obstetrical nurse with a Prussian attitude toward birth, and her docile engineer husband. Sandy lectured us on the female pelvis, fetal anatomy, the stages of labor, how to deal with obstetricians, the pros and cons of hospitals in the area, and a number of topics bearing only peripherally on childbearing. She also held forth on breast feeding, parental roles and responsibilities, and early childhood education. In all, she was colorful, articulate, and rigid—something of an obstetrical Paul Harvey.

The latter half of each two-hour session was devoted to obstetrical calisthenics with our blankets and pillows. The pregnant members of the team (we were ten couples) would lie on their backs around the room and await instructions from ground level. The scene looked like a melon patch in early fall. Under Sandy's tutelage the fathers would then lead their mates through the Lamaze rituals—relaxation exercises and breathing drills. Every now and then we would trade places and I would get to huff and puff (not my best activity) and pretend that a nine-pounder was ramming its head through my pelvis. I assured Judy that I did not need the practice since I had already had a Caesarean delivery through my chest. She didn't find my cancer quips very amusing.

I found it difficult to sit comfortably on the floor,

let alone pant as Judy was instructed to do. I was reminded again of how fortunate it was that she was the reproductive one of the two of us because taxing my body to the extent necessary to deliver a child or even to carry a child was simply not possible. Had our roles been reversed and had Judy suffered the cancer, our family's growth would have been brought to a halt.

Our Lamaze routine was not confined to our evening out. Sandy dictated that we should rehearse our activities daily between classes. Though we played hooky occasionally, we practiced most nights before going to bed. I would time Judy's panting and then describe the nature of a contraction while she undertook the prescribed type of breathing. For amusement we invented a fine vocabulary of contractions to pinpoint the anticipated sensations—a docile contraction, a steadfast pain, a ferocious cramp, a real crotch splitter, or the baby popper itself.

We usually ended our sessions by engaging in the name debate. We had two books that listed thousands of names with their derivations. Doggedly we read through them, giggling at the pomposity of the roots of most names. Occasionally, when one appealed to us or had some familial association, we would jot it down and save it for further discussion. Systematically we narrowed our list until, late one night in early December, with the Lamaze classes now behind us and Judy's belly fairly ready to burst, we concluded that the new baby was really named either Caitlin or Hugh.

In early December, with boot camp over and our names selected, we were ready. Moreover, I had performed my paternal duty of packing the Lamaze bag with lollipops to suck, washcloths to sponge with, a picture for the wall for diversion, extra pillows, and the like. We had the baby's room arranged and Judy's mother joined us once again ready to help out. We had everything in hand except for the baby. Judy's due date, December 15, came and went and Christmas bore down on us with no signs of labor. In addition to the normal tension of anticipation, nagging but unspoken doubts about the status of the pregnancy reappeared in our minds. Could there be something wrong with the baby—this child of life?

Late on the night of December 22, Judy went into labor. She collected her things and I made myself three peanut butter and jelly sandwiches—the final item for the Lamaze sack. It was an odd and wonderful reversal of circumstance to be heading down the Rockville Pike to engage in the ceremony of birth at our old friend the Bethesda Naval Hospital rather than yet another battle in the cancer war. Indeed, Judy would deliver on Tower Four, five floors below my perch, my home away from home, on Tower Nine.

As we pulled up to the hospital, I was chatting excitedly about this and that when I noticed Judy was not responding. When I stopped the car and turned to look at her, I discovered that she was heavily into her breathing patterns with a grimace on her face that told me she was moving quickly past the casual stages of labor. When we finally arrived on the delivery floor, I was dispatched with my bulging Lamaze bag to the "Fathers' Room" while Judy was led away to be examined. I protested that I wanted to stay with her since we were doing Lamaze, but I was rebuffed by a starchy Navy nurse who told me that "rules were rules." We had been told when we inquired months earlier that the Naval Hospital "permitted" natural childbirth and we had not investigated further. As it turned out, John Paul Jones and Dr. Lamaze had never signed a peace treaty—a lesson I was to learn over and over again in the next several hours.

I paced the Fathers' Room for a full thirty minutes waiting for some word on Judy. I was sure she was in active labor and I needed to be with her, since that was essential to our carefully laid game plan. But the Navy felt compelled to keep me quarantined with my sack as a sort of lay leper waiting for my moment of inclusion in the medicalized events taking place in the obstetrical inner sanctums.

Judy had in fact been left alone on an examination table to labor without benefit of any assistance for half an hour until the intern on duty found time to examine her. She performed her solo well, huffing and puffing with each pain and wondering if she was going to deliver by herself. When the intern arrived, a fifteen-second exam confirmed that she was well along in active labor and should be admitted immediately. I was delighted with the news because I assumed it meant we could get on with our teamwork. I was eager to unpack my bag and set into operation the many rituals in which Sandy had drilled us. But that was not, as it turned out, the Navy's way. In an act of humanity, the Navy nurse offered to keep my bag for me but, she explained, I would have to take a fistful of papers to the admissions office to formalize the admission.

"You've got to be kidding," I protested. "My wife's in active labor and you're going to send me to get her papers stamped?"

The Navy nurse, predictably: "Yes, that is a valuable role that fathers perform around here. Someone has to handle the admission and you know all the details, so you can be a big help to your wife and to us." A pause. "Anyway, a rule's a rule."

"C'mon," I whimpered. "We're doing Lamaze. I need to be with her. This is what it is all about. I'll take the papers down afterward. I promise. I'll happily take the papers down afterward."

"Mr. Mullan . . ." she began.

"*Dr.* Mullan," I corrected, hoping it might help.

"Dr. Mullan, this is the time we use to start the IV, shave her, and do the enema. It is time you couldn't be in the room anyway, so please hurry down and get the papers filled out."

"She doesn't need an IV, a shave, or an enema. She didn't have them last time. There is no proven worth to any of them. Anyway"—I paused; I thought I would surely get her on this one—"I've seen an IV or two in my day, ma'am."

"Those are our standing orders, Doctor. There is nothing I can do about it. Now you're wasting time. I suggest you take those papers to the first floor immediately."

Nurse Jones (John Paul?) had me beaten. I took the papers and angrily headed for the elevators.

The scene at the admissions office was grade B comedy. It was now two o'clock in the morning and the single clerk on duty was clearly cowed by my rank and my anger. He tried to move speedily through his paper shuffle, but a variety of things went wrong, redoubling my restlessness. Finally, the computerized typewriter that was to print out multiple copies of the admission forms broke down. The clerk obligingly kicked the machine in strict cliché fashion, and I played my part by slamming copies of *Newsweek* down on the furniture in the waiting room. Eventually, the poor clerk, caught by chance between a broken computer and a crazed Lamaze father, filled out one copy by hand, gave it to me, and promised to bring the rest of the forms to the delivery suite himself.

I sped back to the fourth floor in time to find Judy in the late stages of labor, doing her breathing as well as she could without benefit of coaching, teamwork, or even empathy. Her IV was in place and the razor had done its work. Ritual *über alles.*

I was glad things were progressing quickly but frustrated because we had not been able to work together. Resolutely I began to unpack my sack and prepare the lollipops and washcloths for action. I fantasized some dashing intervention in the labor maneuvers at this point, but Judy was far too well into labor for me to do much. The intern arrived in the room to tell us that her regular obstetrician was on his way to the hospital. His examination at that point, however, found that she was ready to deliver, and he immediately had her taken to the delivery room. I was sent to the men's room to get into a set of green surgical pajamas. I had hardly unpacked my Lamaze bag and the delivery was under way. I felt cheated. Worse yet, I had no idea of what Judy felt, since I had hardly seen her from the beginning of her labor.

The graveyard shift in the delivery room was a nice enough group. Happily, Nurse Jones was not among them since her domain apparently ended at the labor rooms. She was most likely goading and abusing a newly arrived set of parents-to-be. The intern had summoned his resident, for it had become apparent that the baby had no respect for Navy or medical protocol and was going to arrive before Judy's obstetrician made it in from his home.

The delivery room did afford us fifteen minutes of real teamwork. Judy was deeply engaged in the final great act of pregnancy—pushing the infant through the now fully dilated cervix down the birth canal and out into the world. This stage of labor, for which she had trained so rigorously, is one in which the woman can fully drive the events. Capturing each rending contraction, Judy would purse her lips, grit her teeth, and bear down. Two and sometimes three gasping breaths were necessary to squeeze the benefit out of each long cramp. I stuffed pillows behind her back and jacked her into a sitting position with each contraction. She said almost nothing, resting between contractions and conserving her energy for the final thrusts while I barked encouragement throughout like some overwrought high school coach. The cyclic changes in the color of her face as the contractions continued were striking. Resting, she was ashen. As her musculature contorted in exertion at the beginning of a contraction, her face became a flush red, while the wrinkles of her grimace were outlined in white. By the end of a long contraction there were undertones of blue where the red flush had been and finally her face turned pale again with her moments of rest. Judy was truly laboring, a beautiful and disciplined machine.

The final event came quickly. "She's crowning," announced the resident at the end of a long contraction. The next cramp and a monumental heave from Judy produced a greasy, bloody head with matted hair in the resident's hands. But the infant's body did not continue its worldward journey in simple fashion as it should have; for a brief, dramatic moment, the action stopped. A quick check by the resident revealed that the umbilical cord was wrapped twice around the baby's neck, preventing any further movement and simultaneously tourniqueting the as yet unbreathing infant's umbilical blood supply. I don't think Judy realized what was happening, but I did and I was horrified as only a too-well-informed father might be. I wanted to yell, "Cut the thing, goddamnit. Cut it. Cut the goddamned cord!"

Fortunately, my silent instruction was unnecessary. No slouch, the resident already had his probing fingers wedged between the infant's jaw and Judy's underside. He quickly applied two clamps to the taut umbilical cord and cut it between them. He unraveled the strangulating cord and the infant gasped, cried, and passed out of the birth canal into his waiting hands. The suspense was over. It was Caitlin and she was howling magnificently.

No one in that delivery room aside from me and Judy had any notion of the special import of Caitlin's birth. She was a denial of death, of cancer, of debility. For a wild moment in the midst of my jubilation I thought about ripping off my green scrub shirt and showing everybody my monstrous scar. "Caitlin was born in spite of this," I would have said. "Caitlin didn't pay any attention to this. Caitlin doesn't care about chemotherapy or radiation, about paralyzed diaphragms or metastases or recurrences. Caitlin is life, our life, my life. She doesn't care if they try to retire me or give me last rites or any of that. She is here in spite of it all!" I would have thumped my chest victoriously.

Instead, I hugged Judy and did my best to look over and around stethoscope- and syringe-bearing nurses who were hovering over our new daughter. At about that point Judy's obstetrician arrived wearing his full Navy blue uniform. The time was 3:30 a.m. It struck me as strange, though terribly proper, that he would don his uniform for a middle-of-the-night delivery. It occurred to me that if he had slipped on pants and a sweater he might have arrived in time for the birth.

In any event, we were glad of his arrival because he packed sufficient authority to help us circumvent yet one more Navy rule. Judy, who had now been stitched back together, wished to suckle Caitlin for a brief get-acquainted session. She had done this following Meghan's delivery and it had been an important event in both our minds ever since. Caitlin was obviously robust and healthy (she weighed in at 9 pounds 3 ounces) and was ready to suckle. Hospital rules forbade such behavior. The baby was to be sent immediately to the nursery for further examination and cleaning. We protested and appealed to Judy's obstetrician. Middle of the night though it was, his mind was clear on Navy regulations. The rule was that the baby must be sent immediately to the nursery. It was a good rule and he would uphold it. I was sure Nurse Jones liked his style.

The next evening Judy's mother and I went out to dinner together to celebrate. We were both very happy for Judy, for Caitlin, and for ourselves. On Christmas Day, Judy was still in the hospital with Caitlin. Predictably, Navy rules forbade children from visiting the nursery. Nonetheless, we conspired to give Meghan a first peak at her baby sister as a special Christmas present. The elevator on Tower Five, the nursery floor, opened directly across from the plate-glass baby-viewing window. Meghan's head reached only the bottom of the window when she stood on tiptoes. It required no great acrobatics for her to hide beneath the window while the unsuspecting nurse rolled the baby Caitlin over for inspection by the admiring adults. As soon as the nurse had returned to her duties elsewhere, Meghan's nose appeared above the glass for its first sibling confrontation. She was delighted. We retreated as we had come.

The day after Christmas I went alone to the Naval Hospital to bring our new family home. It was a mid-Atlantic winter day, gray, damp, and snowless. I was proud and excited as any father might have been. Moreover, I felt normal. For the moment, the cancer was forgotten and I was doing what any young man with a new baby daughter would do. Judy's mother had the bassinet ready at home. I had my camera in hand and the car packed with extra baby blankets and a pile of clothes for Judy. We said goodbye to Judy's roommates and the nurses and loaded her flowers and Christmas presents into the car. She paused with Caitlin in her arms on the front steps of the National Naval Medical Center. I retreated into the street with my camera in an attempt to record Judy, Caitlin, and the Tower Building all at once. The effort was a failure. Judy and Caitlin were barely recognizable miniatures while the Tower Building loomed massive and overbearing behind them.

Driving home, we had reason to reflect how far we

had come. Only twelve months before, I had been a robust country doctor, still three months from the conception of Caitlin. In the year that had passed, we had encountered the cancer and at least battled it to a standoff. Incredibly, we had used the same precise time to bring forth a new child, a spectacular event that affirmed life and thumbed its nose at cancer and death. In the winter of 1976, a year after I had become a cancer patient, my future remained uncertain. I continued to be bitter about what had happened to me and the burden it had laid on my life. But, whatever the outcome, I had been fulfilled on at least one count—I *had* lived to see my child born. I had shared life with Caitlin. In my own cosmos, that was monumentally important.

CHAPTER

4

Recalled

In September 1975, five months after my initial diagnosis, I was ready to start back to work. Since I
was no longer living in New Mexico and since my
physical energy was circumscribed, neither my old
job at La Clínica nor clinical medicine in general
was a real possibility for me. The Director of the
National Health Service Corps, whose headquarters
were in Rockville, Maryland, was a good friend who
had followed my situation closely. He offered to put
me back to work in an administrative capacity in his
office, tempering the job to my energies. I accepted
happily.

The first day was horrible. I had no clothes that fit
me. It was one thing to loll around the house in
baggy trousers and shirts hopelessly stooped at the
shoulders, but it was another to enter the competi-

tive world of office workers looking like a refugee. I had intended to work only until noon, but by mid-morning I felt ill and my head was swimming. I escaped to the cubicle assigned me to rest my head on the desk until I had sufficient energy to plot my trip home. In a matter of months I had gone from being a physician in charge of La Clínica to being a skeletal new boy posing none too convincingly as a federal bureaucrat. I was very disoriented.

Things did improve. The members of the National Health Service Corps office staff were warm and considerate with me and made my orientation comfortable. No one questioned my part-time schedule and my slow rate of work. Little by little I began to learn my way around. I was given a dictating machine, and memo writing came easily to me. I quickly perceived the critical nature of such items as photocopiers, travel budgets, contract funds, and access to the boss. My experience as a real, live practicing doc turned out to be a unique commodity around the office and useful in a number of ways. I could speak with insight about what it was like to be a National Health Service Corps physician, about the practice of medicine, and about medical training. My new-found usefulness proved to be an essential factor in helping me reestablish my identity as worker, bread-winner, and doctor.

Week by week I became more enthusiastic about the job. I continued to work half a day, returning home for rest in the afternoon. The more involved I became with work, the healthier I felt in my mind, although my body clearly would have found it impossible to work all day. But stepping out of the interesting and preoccupying world of work and climbing into bed for a nap was not as simple or as luxurious as it might sound. For me, afternoon napping became a symbol of my illness. I would lie in a half-darkened room listening to the cheerful noises on the street and be reminded again that I was ill—and that my body might well be gestating more tumor as I lay there. My anxiety was worse in bed than it ever was when I was up and around. My sleep was fitful and I would rejoin the world of the living in the late afternoon feeling tired and tense.

I found it terribly hard during this time to obey my body's needs even though my strength was severely limited. I craved normal activities since I felt I could put the most distance between myself and the disease when I was behaving as if it didn't exist. When I had to acknowledge its presence and effects, I easily became anxious and depressed.

My strength improved steadily, though, and I began to spend more and more time at work. I passed the evenings rewriting the final chapters of *White Coat, Clenched Fist*, the autobiographical account of my political activities during medical school, internship, and residency, which was due to be published as soon as I could finish it. Significantly, however, my redraft of those last chapters was considerably less flamboyant than the initial version had been. I toned down and hedged my claims about the importance of student unrest for the future of the medical profession. One reviewer subsequently called them "dour." One publication, which had considered excerpting portions of the book, wrote my publisher to say that the book's conclusions were too "downbeat" for their audience.

My cancer definitely affected my writing. When I could speak with such little certainty about my own body, how could I make claims about the world at large? My confidence had been hobbled by my disease. Everything I said was far more tentative and judicious than it might have been, and the result undeniably was "downbeat."

Nevertheless, work went well and by January 1976, shortly after Caitlin's birth and four months after I had started back part-time, I was at it full-time again. In March of that year I was put in charge of recruitment for the NHSC.

Throughout this period I was pursued by a nagging expectation. I anticipated being a different person after what I had been through. I had come so close to death that I imagined my perspective on life would be different. I fantasized that certain personal pettinesses of mine would disappear and that I would now be wiser and more temperate than I had been before. My experiences, I reasoned, should have given me new insight and, now that I was recovered, things would be different.

Much to my dismay, things were not different. As far as I could tell, I responded and behaved much as I always had. I was neither missionary nor saint. The egocentricities that had been mine a year earlier had survived the ordeal intact. My personality was alive and passably well, but it was definitely not "born again."

Every month for the year following my hospital discharge, I had to return to the clinic for a chest X-ray and ongoing chemotherapy. Both procedures were punishing. No matter how well I had insulated myself with the concerns of work and home, my monthly pilgrimage to the Oncology Clinic would remind me of the tenuous nature of my "cure."

The most likely point of recurrence for the tumor would be in my chest. My regular reappearance at the Radiology Department never became less frightening. The waiting lines there usually gave me an hour or more to focus on the reason for my visit. Generally unnerved, I would finally enter the X-ray room to be greeted by a technician who knew me well. "How's it going, Doc?" he would always ask. "I don't know. You tell me," I would jokingly reply.

When the films were developed he would hand them to me to carry back to the oncologist in the clinic. I knew as much as anyone about X-rays and easily could have examined my own on the way back to the clinic. I never did. The possibility that I would again discover trouble in my chest was so horrifying to me that it quenched my curiosity. I dutifully returned the unexamined films to the cancer specialist for his perusal. Month after month the X-ray remained stable, a tiny victory each time.

My reward for a good X-ray was another dose of chemotherapy. Relieved to have passed the toughest diagnostic hurdle, I would immediately, even cheerfully, report to the treatment room. There the doctor would carefully prepare two syringes of antitumor agent and methodically administer them through an intravenous needle. I never grew accustomed to the notion that I was willingly accepting toxins into my body. No amount of intellectual reinforcement about the necessity for the treatment made the deliberate use of poison in the body seem reasonable. Set against a lifetime of efforts to stick with healthy foods, to avoid rattlesnakes, jellyfish, and poison ivy, to take vitamins, and to eat liver and spinach, my monthly submission to doses of certified cell-killers seemed absurd.

Moreover, I cooperated with the certain knowledge that twenty-four hours later I would feel wretched. By the next afternoon the nausea and malaise would sweep over me, and for the better part of a week I would struggle with my stomach and my head until mercifully the sensation of acute illness merged into my general aches and pains. Three weeks then remained until the chest X-ray would begin the cycle again.

These three weeks, though, did grant me a period of time during which I could function normally. It amazed me to look in the mirror and, aside from a slight thinness to my hair and ten still-missing pounds, to see a healthy, even robust thirty-three-year-old. In spite of what I had been through and in spite of what I felt like, I looked pretty good. I always expected to see an escapee from Dachau staring back at me out of the mirror. I was no grayer or more lined than I had been before. No one would have had any idea what I had been through if he did not know.

Nonetheless, my body and my mind troubled me. As happy as I was with my new fatherhood and returning to work, in quiet moments there was always time to wonder how things were going—was this ache or that cough a danger sign? The whole idea of "health" became frightfully elusive to me. Not only did I have residual discomforts from all the therapies but the recurrent cycles of chemotherapy caused a host of bodily complaints that—to a one—raised for me the possibility of the return of cancer.

Uncertain as my body was, my mind was in many ways less predictable. I coaxed myself regularly to ignore the minor problems I suffered and to think positively about my body and the future. Sometimes that worked. Often it did not and, even after I had completed the extended course of chemotherapy, I found it hard not to be pessimistic about my state of health. Little things would suddenly trip me up. One evening in a beautiful setting at an open-air concert at Wolf Trap Farm, I coughed and felt a new pain in my chest. The concert was over for me. The music, the people, the setting all faded into the background as I wrestled with a terrible onrush of anxiety. This pain, like so many others, faded out in time. Fortunately other aches proved less devastating mentally, but I never knew what to expect. Even as I careened through these swings of perception, I was frustratingly aware of what was going on. I thought about what a fickle and inaccurate gauge of the body the mind can be. For instance, in Santa Fe prior to the chance chest X-ray, my sense of health was totally intact despite the fact that, in reality, I was extremely ill. After my many cancer treatments, I found it difficult to think of myself as healthy at all, although from a medical point of view my prognosis was much improved.

The mind and body are not only intertwined; in my experience they were often totally indistinguishable. Frequently, after a period of relative well-being, I would wake in the morning feeling ill. Ill, though, wasn't anything as simple as discovering a rash or an elevated temperature. Ill most often meant feeling pokey, subpar, a bit nauseated, or just a little flimsy. If anxiety wasn't part of the symptomatology, it quickly added itself to the brew. Was I upset and worried about my life and health and therefore feeling rocky or was it the reverse—was I physically ill with some old or new manifestation of my disease and did worry, reasonably enough, come as a result of that? Much of the time I had no idea what was going on. Fitz, I would tell myself, you're highstrung and jumpy and are making yourself suffer needlessly. There's nothing wrong with you except a slight and persistent case of fear. Having decided therefore that I was neurotic rather than terminal, I would breathe a little easier because, like most people, I would rather be a little hypochondriacal than a little cancerous.

My sense of relief would usually last a few minutes until the next bout of malaise would sweep over me. Then I would haul out thermometers, aspirins, and antacids in the hope that I was only a little bit sick—a touch of flu, a bit of a cold, maybe an early strep throat. Occasionally the onset of an incidental illness was indeed the culprit. A fellow cancer patient has described it as the "Goody-it's-the-flu Syndrome." No one is quite so happy as a cancer patient when the nonspecific yuks turn out to be something delightfully insignificant like a bout of viral diarrhea or a good chest cold. The relief of being able to put a name and a good prognosis on a set of vague symptoms is a joy that I came to appreciate.

The return to apparent health and my hearty appearance, however, created a new dilemma. While I had no desire to flaunt my cancer, it was the overwhelming event of the previous year and, in some ways, of my entire life. As I became active again professionally and socially I would meet people whom I had known previously. It was impossible to know how to respond to the simple query "How have you been?" The answer "Fine" was not true. "Pretty good, other than a touch of cancer," didn't work either. While I was not averse to sharing my experiences, I had neither the time nor the energy to share my tale with casual acquaintances.

In the course of normal events Judy or I would be asked frequently, "What brings you to the Washington area?" or "Why are you working here?" Those questions all had a simple answer, but it was one that invited a degree of detail and intimacy for which we were not always prepared. We both bobbed and weaved in our responses depending upon the circumstances and our frame of mind. Behind the problem, however, lurk questions for anyone who has had a serious illness: How do you integrate the sickness into your ongoing life? How do you acknowledge it without dwelling on it? And how do you put it behind you without denying it?

Without discussing it much, Judy and I groped along, telling some people, avoiding it with others, responding to questions when asked but making as little of it as we could. Meghan talked about my "Yaya" freely, which we supported. At one point when we were signing a contract to buy a new house, the real estate agent, who knew of my illness, admonished me to keep Meghan quiet. Meghan had apparently given the owner of the house a long and detailed account of "Daddy's Yaya," jeopardizing, the agent was sure, the house closing. As it turned out, we settled on the house without any hitches, but my illness remained alive for everybody in the family.

Sports had always been part of my life and my identity. Now that I had some strength back I began to experiment with my body to find out what it could bear in the way of athletics. Basketball had been my favorite sport. My first efforts at playing proved disappointing, since my arms were extremely weak and my chest and neck were so tight that I had trouble looking at the basket when I stood close to it. I had never realized how much time on the basketball court is spent looking up. When I was far enough back so I could see the basket easily, I wasn't strong enough to shoot the ball that far, and when I was in close enough so I could shoot, I had trouble seeing the basket. I played some pickup games with grade-school kids and found that level of play well tuned to my strength. I was more of a coach, I realized, than a competitor.

Tennis and squash were also particular favorites. While I knew that I did not have the strength yet for a full-fledged competition, I visited a squash court at a local club several times to find out what I could do with a racquet. To my delight it turned out that my swing was unimpeded and I could hit away on the forehand and the backhand almost as if my chest had never been pulled apart. The joy of hitting the ball those few times was tremendous. I let myself fantasize that people were in the gallery watching me, admiring my strokes. They could not possibly know, I gloated, that I was a cancer patient not yet a year beyond surgery. No one was watching but I felt as good as if they had been.

My physical limitations created the sensation of a strangely accelerated aging process that left my shell looking thirty-three years old while turning my insides into those of an octogenarian. I hoped that there was more to come in the way of regained strength and endurance, but I was sure that my physical clout was permanently diminished. When I heard friends, now in their thirties, bemoan their shortness of breath or their beer bellies, I found myself far less sympathetic than I might have been a short time before. The incremental demands of age, the steady pickpocketing that happens to us all, seemed nothing compared to the Brink's robbery that had been performed on my body. What's a little flab on the waist or droop in the breast, I thought often, compared to a permanently hijacked lung.

My problems, though, when they struck, came from things I hadn't even thought about. Dr. Mills had been checking me periodically from his surgical perspective. In May 1976, fourteen months after my diagnosis and surgery, he noted a pin-sized hole that never had healed in the middle of the scar running down my sternum. Most of the time it was covered with a scab that would occasionally slough off and drain a small quantity of yellow fluid. In his office one day he took a sterile probe and slipped it into the opening to determine its depth. To my surprise more than half an inch of the probe disappeared into me without any sensation.

"We had better find out what is going on inside there," he announced, and sent me to the Radiology Department. There the radiologist inserted a tiny plastic catheter, which disappeared even farther inside me than the probe had. The radiologist then pumped contrast fluid into the aperture. When it began to leak out, he stopped and X-rayed my mid-chest from a number of different angles.

Dr. Mills shared the results with me later that afternoon. There was a large, infection-filled cavity in my sternum which was undoubtedly a result of the surgery and subsequent intensive radiation. The sternum would need to be opened and cleaned out in the hopes that it would heal from the inside out. More tumor was unlikely but not impossible.

Judy was depressed at the turn of events. I argued with her, playing my stiff-upper-lip role, that things could have been a lot worse. The basic diagnosis, after all, was infection and not cancer. "And what's a little infection?" I asked cavalierly. A simple surgical cleansing of my sternum, I pointed out patiently, was a small, curative procedure that would leave me with nothing worse than a funny-looking scar in the middle of my chest. A date was set for surgery. The weekend before the operation, Memorial Day, 1976, we traveled to Chincoteague, Virginia, with our good friends the Kindigs, who had shared many of our ups and downs. We lolled about the beach in the late-spring warmth and watched the children play in the sand. Dave and I talked about our futures and our ambitions. I was sure that a week on Tower Nine was the worst that awaited me and that I would recover quickly. The late-May surf was still frigid but it felt good to me. I led the group into the breakers, feeling strong and healthy for the first time in many months and, as it turned out, for the last time for many more.

    Three days after surgery I left the hospital with a small bandage plugging a walnut-sized hole in my chest. The procedure had gone well and I had no reason to second-guess my optimism. Two weeks later, however, the wound showed no signs of healing. In fact, it gave every indication of being reinfected. The surgeons tried antibiotics and a number of different soaps and dressings, to no avail. By the time another two weeks had gone by, I had begun to lose weight and feel chronically weak and nauseated. The conclusion was that more infection was lurking within the breastbone and further surgery was indicated to remove it. So again I moved into Tower Nine, this time to have the walnut-sized excavation in my sternum hollowed out to the size of an egg. I was home again and back trying to work within several days, but the infection reemerged almost immediately. In fact, Dr. Mills had determined at surgery that much of my sternum was invaded by small channels of infection. The intensive radiation delivered to the center of my chest had all but killed my breastbone. Left as it was with a pocket of contamination following the initial surgery and scalded as it had been with therapeutic radiation, the breastbone was totally unable to defend itself against the weak but persistent bacteria burrowing within it. The result was the slowly emerging infection that I had dismissed casually only a month before.

The obvious question was what to do. Dr. Mills counseled patience as well as a consultation with a plastic surgeon. Plastic surgery had always seemed to me to be a frivolous medical specialty and I had never expected to draw on the services of a plastic surgeon. Dr. Mills asked Dr. Diane Colgan to his office to examine me. Dr. Colgan was attractive, earnest, and my age, give or take a year. She quietly studied the X-rays, examined my chest, and discussed the options available if the infection would not heal by itself. The possibilities were elaborate and lengthy and, to a one, sufficiently treacherous to dismiss all of the bravado with which I had recently approached this non-cancer in my breastbone.

She and Dr. Mills advised a conservative course continuing with local cleansing and antibiotics in the hopes of getting the chest to heal by itself. In the meantime, however, an alternative form of therapy was suggested. Over the years the Navy had experimented with hyperbaric oxygen therapy for a variety of medical problems. Biological events at pressures greater than normal were of obvious interest to the Navy, since life beneath the waves was lived under hyperbaric conditions. High-pressure oxygen treatment for indolent infections had intrigued surgeons and infectious-disease experts for some time. The principle of the treatment was to increase the oxygen content of the environment (a chamber) to 100 percent (as opposed to the 20 percent found in room air). The pressure of the oxygen would then be increased to three atmospheres. Pure oxygen under pressure was felt to promote rapid wound healing since the oxygen content of both the wound and the circulating blood was greatly increased. Reports published in the mid-1970s suggested that infections such as mine—technically known as osteoradionecrosis—responded well to extended hyperbaric oxygen treatment and could indeed be cured.

I didn't like the idea much since it was time-consuming, experimental, and cumbersome. Moreover, high concentrations of oxygen had occasionally caused a form of pulmonary toxicity, a complication I could ill afford. Yet the alternative—immediate major, risky surgery—was no bargain either. So one afternoon late in July 1976, shortly after the nation had celebrated its 200th anniversary and I had limped through my thirty-fourth, I reported to the basement of a laboratory building in back of the National Naval Medical Center. I had no idea what to expect and fantasized a gymnasium equipped with a massive diving bell. I imagined that I might climb inside and sit on the hard bench with a towel across my lap like some jock in a sauna while I was treated to hyperbaric magic.

The treatment was, in fact, fairly sensational but not at all as I had imagined it. To be sure, the lab did have some large chambers with swinging doors and multiple metal rivets but they were not for me. The chief petty officer who greeted me, a savvy veteran of submarine duty and naval research, introduced me to my own personal landlocked bathysphere. My chamber was an eight-foot-long horizontal cylinder made of clear plastic almost an inch thick. A stretcher on which I was to lie rolled neatly into the cylinder and a bulkhead was swung shut and locked behind me to seal the contraption. The gas composition inside the tube and the internal pressure were controlled by a remote console. My sentence in the chamber was an hour and a half a day, five days a week.

Whatever my imagined sauna might have been like, the claustrophobia in the tube promised to be unpleasant. I consoled myself that I would be able to do a great deal of reading. Wrong again. The high concentration of oxygen made the chamber potentially combustible. Therefore, everything within it, save, I supposed, my body, had to be fireproof. The sheets and pillow on the stretcher as well as the pajama bottoms I was given were made of special material. Books and magazines were forbidden since, the chief petty officer pointed out, paper burns well.

To combat boredom, if not downright craziness, a 24-inch color TV was planted in the wall next to the cylinder and the bulkhead was wired for sound. With what was left of my sense of adventure, dressed only in faded, fireproof pajama bottoms, I climbed onto the stretcher and was rolled into my hyperbaric tube. The bulkhead was swung shut and locked, leaving me in a tiny, silent, plastic world. The chief petty officer and his crew chatted with me through the sound system and explained their every maneuver in advance. First I would hear a hissing noise, which was the oxygen being pumped in and room air being removed. Next, and rather dramatically, they explained that they were "taking me down"—Navy talk, as I learned, for running the pressure up. My ears would pop and feel funny, they warned, on the way "down" as well as on the way back "up." I should chew and yawn a good deal. After a few minutes they told me that I was "on the bottom" and should make myself comfortable for the duration. For my amusement they turned on the TV.

I had a choice of soap operas or game shows, neither of which I found entertaining. I tried sleeping, but it was difficult both because the stretcher was uncomfortable and because I wasn't used to napping in daylight with people watching. So I spent a good deal of time looking at my exquisitely pink fingertips (thanks to the high concentration of oxygen in my blood) and worrying about what all that oxygen might be doing to damage my one functioning lung.

Doggedly I pursued the treatment. Every afternoon through the heavy hot days of August I showed up for therapy. The chief petty officer and his men courteously took me down and brought me up again. While I was "under," the staff cleaned equipment, did paperwork, and played cards. They were businesslike technicians who knew a fair bit about diving chambers but nothing about seminoma or bone infections. Regularly they asked me, the doctor, about the patient. The patient, my chest, was not doing very well. The wound showed no signs of healing and continued to fester. After three weeks of hyperbaric oxygen treatment Dr. Colgan and Dr. Mills agreed to abandon the effort and move to plastic surgery.

Although I understood that it was a reasonable suggestion made by reasonable people trying to find a solution to a tough problem, the idea seemed grotesque to me. Hadn't I done my penance? Hadn't I had my cancer and licked it? Hadn't I borne its sequelae and accepted the loss of a lung? Hadn't I been willing to go back to surgery to get a final pothole fixed? Why was the punishment to continue? Why was my upper body now to be cannibalized in a painful and disfiguring assault that at best would get me back to where I had been *after* the cancer? Why?

Dr. Colgan had devised an ambitious scheme for solving my problem. She had concluded that my breastbone in almost its entirety was rotten and would have to be removed. The skin overlying it and some of the tissue beneath it were likewise damaged by radiation and infection and would have to be sacrificed as well. I didn't need to call on my medical training to envision the postcard-sized rectangular hole this would leave in the middle of my chest. Since the heart and lungs lie immediately beneath the sternum and clearly need a protective cover, the obvious question was how to reconstruct the front of my chest.

Drs. Colgan and Mills agreed that my rib cage would keep my thorax in place well enough so that no structural replacement would be necessary for the breastbone itself. What was needed was a sufficient amount of flesh to fill in the hole, cushion the structures beneath, and provide protective skin to the entire area. Enter the plastic surgeon.

Dr. Colgan's plan was this: At an initial operation she would elevate a skin flap on the right side of my belly. This meant that she would detach three sides of a large rectangle of skin and fat on my flank. The fourth side, the side closest to the midline of my abdomen, would remain attached. This was to be the skin that would eventually cover the chest. In order to move it there, however, she had to plant it in some location that could continue to nurture it while it was moved.

And so the surgery passed from the commonplace to the extraordinary. She would take the second side of the skin flap—the one opposite the side that remained attached to my abdomen—and sew it to an exposed surface on my right forearm. This procedure was not intended as a ghoulish exercise in body transplants but rather as a method to provide a second blood supply to the belly tissue that would at this point be suspended between the right arm and the right side of the abdomen. In a matter of weeks the right arm would develop a rich system of blood flow into the flank tissue such that, at a second operation, the fourth side of the skin flap—the side still attached to the abdomen—could be severed. The flap, now supported totally by the arm, could be swung into place over the chest. The plan called for the removal of the breastbone and its adjacent tissues at that second operation, with the skin flap moved into place and sewed down immediately following the removal of the diseased tissue. The skin flap would remain attached to the arm for several weeks after the second operation to ensure a continued blood supply while it established new channels of blood flow into the surrounding tissues of the chest. When that had been accomplished, the flap would be detached from the arm. The final side of the flap would be permanently sewed in place and the skin on the arm would be sutured closed, leaving only a scar.

In all, it wasn't a good way to spend the rest of the Bicentennial summer, but there weren't many options. Dr. Mills and Dr. Colgan were persuasive and reassuring in their discussions and recommendations. Dr. Mills kindly offered me my old room back on Tower Nine. Dr. Colgan's gentle, evenhanded, slightly military manner that I came to know well over the next months appealed to me. I accepted their counsel.

Mom and Dad, who had just left for a vacation in England, flew home. Judy girded herself for another stint of single parenthood, Meghan drew me a gallery of pictures to decorate my hospital room, and in mid-August I moved back onto Tower Nine.

The first operation went well, although the sensation of awakening with my arm sewn to my side and vice versa was bizarre. The whole area was bundled in bandages and carried in a sling. Belatedly I discovered that I wasn't very good at eating, brushing my teeth, or combing my hair left-handed, though I was to learn rapidly. Writing was pretty much out of the question. My chest continued to fester and required an elaborate set of dressings itself. Between that and my skin flap, the corpsmen on Tower Nine spent hours of effort and cartons of bandages keeping me properly dressed. In early September I underwent the second operation—the big one. Dr. Mills presided over the removal of my sternum, while Dr. Colgan saw to the implantation of the rectangular patch of skin and fat from my side into my chest. I awoke with my arm scrunched flat across the middle of my chest and massive quantities of gauze bandaging everything from my chin to my hip bones. I looked like half a mummy. Additionally, the fronts of both my thighs had been skinned by a microtome—a plastic surgeon's bologna slicer—to remove tiny strips of skin which were then used to cover the pit on the side of my belly where the skin flap had been detached. These lox-like strips would produce a protective layer of tough skin over the wound. The donor areas on my thighs would regenerate by themselves with good care.

Dr. Mills and Dr. Colgan were satisfied with the operation. They had had to remove more skin and bone than they had anticipated, but Dr. Colgan's generous flap had been more than sufficient to cover it. Now it was up to my body to heal for all it was worth—to heal the new patchwork on the chest, to heal the pit on my right flank where the flap had come from, and to heal the donor sites on my legs. My major responsibility at this point was to submit to endless bandaging, unbandaging, and rebandaging by the ever-present, ever-faithful Navy corpsmen.

John Marcus was a corpsman who took special care of me. Even though he called me "Dr. Mullan" throughout and I always called him "Marcus," we shared an intimacy from the start. Not only did he carry out my bandaging and personal care with skill and ingenuity (he improved on the bandaging procedures designed by the doctors) but he nurtured my ribald, adolescent side. A young man who liked women, motorcycles, and skin diving (in that order), he always had an off-color story or a rowdy incident to share with me. At a time when I felt very distant from levity and youthfulness, Marcus spoke to me like a locker-room buddy, treating me to a brand of gentle male jocularity that was wonderfully affirming. It felt good to guffaw at a randy escapade or a plain old dirty joke. Yet Marcus wasn't all bawdy. He loaned me a lovely book of poems and made cartoon-like sketches of some of the more outlandish things I fantasized doing—in frustration—to the hospital equipment and routine. He made me laugh at a time when laughing was becoming more and more difficult.

The wound would not heal. Slowly at first, but then in increasing quantity, the drainage from under the skin flap turned to pus. After a week of routine efforts Dr. Colgan tried a more aggressive scheme—dripping a sterilizing solution from an IV bottle through a long tube planted underneath the top of my new chest cover. A rubber drainage tube was placed under the skin at the bottom of the flap and was attached to a suction machine to extract all of the sterilizing fluid as well as any pus present. Day and night the suction pump ran. I felt like an incidental human way station on the Alaska pipeline. The noise, mess, and discomfort of the entire scheme were oppressive. I had a fantasy of destruction. I would arise from my bed without my tubes, heave the bottle of fluid against the wall, and take the IV pole and smash the suction pump into scrap metal. Whatever living out the fantasy might have done to relations with the hospital staff, I realized it was unachievable with only one arm available, my left one at that.

After several weeks of suction-pump heroics and general frustration, Dr. Colgan took me back to the operating room. She removed the drains and opened the rectangular patch of skin along its bottom border in order to clean it and pack it with bandages. This was to be the new strategy for healing. My arm remained attached to my chest throughout, since there was no way to be sure that the skin graft was getting adequate blood supply from the adjacent tissue yet.

The months that followed were terrible ones for

me. Methodically, four times a day, the corpsmen unpacked and repacked the festering tunnel under the skin patch. Dr. Colgan tried irrigating with this solution and that. Very little progress was made. To make matters worse, Dr. Colgan departed for several weeks of vacation, leaving me in the hands of a generally befuddled staff.

September became October. Judy enrolled Meghan in a parent co-op nursery and brought me tales of new friends and new achievements. I watched the leaves turn from green to yellow to brown out the window of Tower Nine with no sense that I would ever return to the outside world. I was a captive of technology gone awry—a victim of a iatrogenic, or medically caused, illness. While the therapy had apparently licked the cancer, it had destroyed my anterior chest. One treatment begot another and, in an effort to patch the chest, my side had been transplanted upwards with the assistance of my arm. Now, arm stuck to side, side stuck to chest, and chest refusing to heal. I was an iatrogenic catastrophe.

I had hour upon hour, day after day, to ponder my predicament. Time and again my thoughts returned to the mediastinal biopsy on that fateful Good Friday a year and a half before. If that biopsy had gone well, my chest would never have been opened. If my chest had not been cracked, my lungs would never have been damaged—save for the minimal effects of radiation—and my sternum would never have become infected. In short, I would have survived the cancer with minimal physical punishment. Instead I was embroiled in a second, harrowing fight for my life which was inescapably linked to the errant biopsy. That circumstance, that bald fact, haunted me, cycling and recycling uselessly but compellingly through my consciousness.

That first surgery became a symbol for me of everything I found objectionable about life in a medical center. Time and again I was reminded of the awkwardness of the human being—me—in the hospital. I was a bad fit, a seven-sided peg in a hexagonal hole. The sicker and the more dependent I was, the more apparent this became, because I had to rely increasingly on the system not only for medical care but for the amenities of life. My well-being rested on physician's orders ("There's nothing ordered for that") or nurses' good humor ("We're too busy to get you up now. Wait a while"). The internal inconsistencies of the hospital, things that had never occurred to me as a doctor, surprised me frequently as a patient. The fine-honed pharmacology of a sleeping pill, for instance, was destroyed by the thoughtless "standing order" for a 2 a.m. temperature check. Likewise, the precision of a calorie-rich dinner prepared especially for my debilitated body by the nutritionists was negated by serving it on hospital time at quarter to five in the afternoon, long before I was the least bit hungry.

Occasionally I encountered real crassness—a physician treating me in a deprecating way or a technician shoving me mindlessly and painfully this way and that for an X-ray. But that didn't happen often. The real problem is that the modern medical center is, by its very nature, depersonalizing. The multiple purposes of the medical center (teaching and research along with patient care) as well as the necessary teams of doctors and constantly rotating shifts of nurses and corpsmen make continuity and intimacy difficult to achieve.

At times, though, the system was surprisingly and wonderfully human. During one period I was cared for by a veteran nurse, a woman who had practiced her profession for more than twenty years and knew it thoroughly. She had five children of her own and a grandchild on the way. I enjoyed her most when she was on the night shift and spent time regaling me with tales of her career and how nursing had changed. Once when I was feeling particularly wretched she gave me a bed bath. When she finished it, she insisted that I spend ten minutes with my feet in a tub of warm water. I demurred at first, but she persisted and I gave in. When I was done, she patted my feet dry and put me back in bed. The relaxation and intimacy of the foot bath left me feeling mellow, pampered, and peaceful in a way that I had not known in many weeks. The foot bath, she explained, was a trick she had learned many years before in nursing school, and she carried on with it even though it was no longer touted as proper nursing practice. She had successfully breached the gap between sci-

ence and my psyche. I felt greatly in her debt and
had her bathe my feet as often as I could after that.

During these weeks of helplessness I read a
lengthy autobiography of Alexander Dolgun called
An American in the Gulag. Dolgun, born in the
United States of Polish parents, moved to the Soviet
Union at the age of ten with his father, a contract
laborer. In 1948, aged twenty-one, he was picked up
by the Soviet Secret Police for alleged spying activities. In the book's 500 pages he details his experiences as an inmate in Russia's worst prisons and
forced-labor camps. Eventually he was released and
managed to return to the United States and record
his tale.

The most gripping sections of the book concern his
interrogation and beatings in two Moscow prisons.
Standard treatment included isolation, starvation,
sleep deprivation, and eighteen hours of interrogation a day. Throughout he had no idea what his
captors were after or what they planned to do with
him, although it became increasingly clear they
cared little whether he died or not. From hour to
hour and day to day he never knew what would
come next, more beatings, more interrogation, new
prisons, new interrogators, or perhaps a respite. No
formal charges were leveled against him, he had no
lawyers or advocates, no visitors, no contact with the
outside world, and there were long periods when he

was allowed to talk to no one except his brutal interrogator.

Using psychological gimmicks, he became colossally resourceful at countering his depression and deprivation. He worked out ingenious systems to steal minutes of sleep. He captured a fly and talked to it incessantly, achieving a sense of companionship. He counted his paces as he stumbled up and down his cell, back and forth to the interrogation rooms, imagining each step was leading him out of Moscow and the Soviet Union and across Europe to the westernmost extremity of Spain, from which he would get to the United States. His ingenuity and staying power in the face of an incomprehensible and capricious calamity were truly fantastic.

I often woke at night with confused thoughts about me and Alexander Dolgun. Our experiences seemed to me strikingly parallel. For the previous year and a half I had been captive of an incomprehensible and capricious disease. It struck me as quickly and unexpectedly as the Secret Police that swept Dolgun off a Moscow street. Furthermore, the course and outcome of my disease remained as unfathomable to me as Dolgun's future did to him during his long captivity. Like Dolgun, I had to modify my life expectations. I had to face the notion of death and, at times, even wished for it. I had to deal with fearsome and ultimately permanent changes in my body which I thought I could never accept. In fact, I discovered capacities and adaptabilities that I never knew I had.

Interrogators and dressing changes, beatings and operations, abuses and procedures. And yet life went on in the belief that there would be escape, relief, freedom. The struggle for me in my medical gulag was never a question of bravery or heroism. Doggedness was what it took to survive—drab, stolid, life-sustaining doggedness.

As the fall wore on I became a fixture once again on Tower Nine. Patients came and went, residents rotated to other services, new nurses joined the staff as old ones left, but I was always there. The corpsmen made an ornate cardboard sign for my door: DOCTOR MULLAN, RESIDENT PHYSICIAN.

During these months on Tower Nine I became a true veteran of the system. I learned to refer to the lower reaches of the hospital as "A Deck" and "B Deck," as they were called in Navy parlance, and the North Wing and South Wing as "Fiveside" and "Sevenside." The clock, too, was Navy, with breakfast served at 0730 and dinner at 1700. Worst of all, though, the day began at 0600 with the corpsmen making rounds to check temperatures and blood pressures and pass out medications. I had real trouble with the 6 a.m. wake-up routine.

But, like a canny old inmate of a state penitentiary, I did the best I could to bend the many rules to my own ends, so that life, in its way, became more comfortable. First of all, my room was off to one side of the main corridor and was easily skipped by the busy corpsmen collecting temperatures and blood pressures at the crack of dawn. Trading on this fact, I went to the corpsmen one at a time as they rotated on night duty and suggested that since my decrepit condition was so stable, a 6 a.m. checkup was not necessary. To a person they acquiesced. Next I established a pattern of eating late at almost all meals, so that my breakfast was always taken off the meal cart and put directly on a warmer to await me. Mercifully, at 0730 I was not confronted with Philadelphia scrapple, raisin bran, and eggs over lightly. I took pride in my achievement.

A problem did arise with my scheme. During the first months of this hospitalization two affable and inefficient cleaning women alternated responsibility for the janitorial duties on Tower Nine. Both women were friendly and supportive and always asked how I was doing and how my family was. I learned both of their names and we became friends. Their approach to cleaning Tower Nine was anything but aggressive. They rarely entered a room if a patient was there and never entered if a physician was present. They did succeed in emptying wastebaskets, but mop, dustrag, and vacuum were rarely seen on Tower Nine. I am no stickler for cleanliness, but I had noticed impressive dust balls collecting in the recesses of my room. I wrote them off to friendship.

Suddenly the women disappeared, supplanted by a taciturn, methodical man in his mid-thirties who systematically cleaned the entire floor daily, using mop, rag, and vacuum. The dust balls went but so did the amicable small talk. Jonathan—that was his name—slavishly followed his battle plan day after day like a well-drilled commando on a forward mission. He arrived on the ward at 0700 and began by vacuuming the halls, so that even with my door shut I could hear him coming. He then dispensed with the vacuum and began his room-by-room shakedown. The time was 0715 and my room came first. Why first, I don't know, but Jonathan never varied from his scheme, charted, I am sure, in inner sanctums of the housekeeping department.

He started by knocking on the door, but his knock was no ordinary knock. It made the windowpanes shake and often brought me up on one elbow with the adrenaline running. I would invite him to enter (did I have a choice?) and without the nicety of a hello or good-morning, he began his job. I would sink back in bed, feigning sleep in the hope he would not turn on the lights. He dusted first, scouring invisible dirt from the top of my bedside lamp. He cleaned other items in a random sort of way, but the bedside lamp seemed to be essential to orient him to his mission. It got well scrubbed five times a week. When the dusting was done he turned to the bathroom, banging the door open and giving it a noisy once-over. Finally, there was the wet mop. His weapon was an ancient string affair which surely did no more than redistribute dirt already present. Painstakingly, he worked his way among the tables and chairs and under the bed to ensure the daily rearrangement of bacteria on my floor. In the process he bumped and rattled the bed frequently, which I responded to by repositioning myself, trying to look as pained as possible.

Eventually Jonathan worked his way out of the room, returned his mop to its pail, and moved off down the hall, occasionally remembering to close the door. The time was then 0725. There were nine rooms on the floor. I calculated that at his demonstrated rate he finished the floor by 0845, which explained why he was not around much when I got up sometime after 0800. Those times I did see him, he was either sitting in the janitor's room smoking or wandering around the hospital without particular purpose. He did a proficient if sullen job of caring for Tower Nine, a task he apparently finished in two hours every morning. The rest of the day was his.

I was sufficiently cowed by the man so that I never negotiated with him. My powers of sleep in the early morning proved strong and usually I was comfortable again by 0730, the only recollection of Jonathan being relief that he had gone.

At one point earlier in the course of my treatments, Dr. Mills mentioned to me that he had just operated on a teenager with a chest tumor similar to mine. The boy, he told me, showed no other signs of disease and his surgery had gone well. This information stayed with me, so that one day during my long hospitalization when one of the staff physicians stopped me in the hall and said, "Meet Billy. He's your twin," I knew immediately what she meant. Now Billy was back in the hospital. At a routine checkup the previous week his chest X-ray had revealed a shadow in his right lung. The possibility of a metastasis could not be ignored and he was on the surgical schedule for the next morning.

Billy was a solid, impish fifteen-year-old, the paradigm of a boy-man. That first night of his back in the hospital he padded up and down the ward innumerable times in a Washington Redskins bathrobe. The walls of his room were decorated with Mickey Mouse and John Denver posters, and his bed was littered with stuffed animals given him by his classmates. He was, he reported, a "star" halfback on the junior varsity football team. That evening his girlfriend was visiting him, a pretty girl with braces and a contoured blouse.

Billy was interested in comparing notes and was curious about the history of my skin graft and why my arm was strapped to my side. Yet he had trouble remaining still through our discussion and left frequently to tease the nurses, walk the hall, or flirt with his girlfriend.

The shadow on Billy's lung proved to be more of the tumor and Billy lost his right upper lobe, guaranteeing him a significant pulmonary deficit for the rest of his life and most certainly ending his football career. His recovery on the ward was slow. For ten days he went everywhere with a tube protruding from his chest connected to a portable drainage system. He scowled much of the time and rarely had much of anything to say. Behind his back the corpsmen called him a crybaby and yet his manner was imperious rather than infantile.

Billy was visited frequently by a young man with a crew cut who wore a short jacket with a small but distinctive sharpshooter's emblem on the breast pocket. The man often stood in the hall outside Billy's room chatting with Billy or other patients. His relationship with Billy did not seem particularly close. My guess was that he was an older brother, an uncle, or perhaps a family friend. When I asked Billy who the visitor was, his answer was simple. "That's my dad. He's a Marine. He shoots pistols." Needless to say, I was surprised, because of the man's youth and Billy's apparent lack of interest in him. It turned out he was a master marksman and a pistol instructor in the Marines. He was thirty-four years old—my age.

Billy and his circumstances perplexed me. On many levels we had a great deal in common—similar diseases, physically active lives that were being curtailed . . . young men's cancers. Yet in other ways the gap between us was immense and prevented us from being able to talk candidly about our conditions, a fact I regretted. I was never able to reach out to Billy the way I had with Zwicker during my previous stay on Tower Nine. His very youth made it particularly hard to bridge the gap. I was scared of my disease and would have liked to talk to him about it. But Billy wasn't a good candidate for talk, since his

approach to illness was marked by denial—consis-
tent, effective, teenage denial. The fact that Billy's
tumor had metastasized complicated the situation
because it caused conflicting emotions in me. It
made me fearful, for the obvious reason that it suggested that my tumor might do likewise, and it provided me with a small measure of relief, for I had
managed, thus far, to escape recurrence.

This snarl of sentiment that I felt about Billy left
me with strong feelings about him—feelings of
friendship and alienation, kinship and rivalry, intimacy and distance. When he was discharged from
the hospital, he left without stopping by my room.
Although I have vivid memories of "my twin," I
know nothing more about his life or his illness.

Sometime later in my stay the nurses told me that
I was going to have "company," by which they
meant that another physician was going to be admitted to Tower Nine. Jim Barnes was a thirty-
three-year-old Navy physician with a wife and three
children. He had been a normal, active young man
until, three months before, he suffered a heart attack,
a blow that changed his life. After a lot of thought
and discussion and many medical tests, he decided to
undergo cardiac bypass surgery, a procedure that
would increase the supply of blood to his heart muscle in an effort to avoid further heart attacks. He
came to the National Naval Medical Center to have
the procedure done.

I first saw him sitting on a couch in the hallway reading a book. He wore his lieutenant commander's white uniform, and it struck me as strange that a member of the Navy Medical Corps should be sitting on a couch reading a book instead of a patient's chart. But then I realized, of course, that this wasn't really Barnes the Doctor before me—it was Barnes the Patient. I was also surprised that he was wearing his uniform in the hospital. He was here, after all, on sick leave, it was the day prior to surgery, and there was no necessity for him to be in clothes at all, let alone a uniform. When I thought about it, however, this too made sense. He was responding much as I had. The longer he could be a doctor, a Navy doctor, the longer he was in control of the situation and the longer he was not a patient. Even if he lolled about the ward, a totally uncharacteristic activity for a doctor, he probably felt more comfortable in his doctor outfit.

I noticed him later that day sitting on the same couch in the hall reviewing his medical history with the anesthesiologist who was to put him to sleep the following morning. Again, he was every bit the doctor, precise, seemingly assured, definite about the dosages of the various potent drugs he was taking. He recited a hundred facile facts, ones that he had often collected from patients, for the benefit of the anesthesiologist, who duly marked them on his sheet. He had no allergies, he had had no operations, he drank three cups of coffee a day and smoked a pack and a half of cigarettes. He clung to these facts as definitions of who he was, a reasonable, hard-working, mildly sick thirty-three-year-old man; someone who needed medical care, he would concede, but not a candidate for death.

Later that night I talked to Barnes. I introduced myself, and he said yes, he had heard there was another doctor on the ward. We compared notes about our backgrounds, our training, and our medical conditions. He was quieter than I was, although he wiggled his foot persistently as we talked. I took comfort in telling him about all the surgery I had undergone, trying to reassure him, in a sense, that he too could overcome his illness. In fact, I think I was clinging to my many operations as evidence that I was still alive. I was the old boy. I knew a little bit about the unknown—not much, perhaps, but a hell of a lot more than Barnes did.

Barnes had pushed for coronary angiography, the contrast X-ray study of the heart that would reveal the extent of narrowing of his coronary arteries. The doctors caring for him were not sure he needed this test, but he intervened as a physician and insisted on receiving it. It was the grim information obtained from the angiography that put surgery immediately on his agenda. The result was that his name was placed at the top of the operating schedule for the following morning.

Barnes and his wife and his mother had had a good weekend together. He had checked into the hospital on Friday but spent Saturday and Sunday with them. They had seen Washington, had some good meals, enjoyed themselves. I didn't ask him if he could forget his surgery amidst the levity, but I doubted that he could.

Barnes looked healthy. Of medium height, he was clean-shaven and pudgy. When he put on his short bathrobe, he looked like a veteran prizefighter walking around the ward with his knees showing. He did not appear sick. In fact, I don't know if "sick" is really the right word to describe his condition. Rather he was precarious, at risk, close to the edge. So much of him looked so good, and yet the malfunction of three tiny pipes deep in his body, the coronary arteries, threatened to stop his machine and steal his life at any moment. That is a strange kind of sickness, but it is very real and Barnes had it.

His children were aged seven, four, and two. He told me that the seven-year-old boy had asked him spontaneously before he left home if Daddy might die when he went for his operation. We smiled nervously at one another and didn't pursue the topic. I remembered that Meghan had asked Judy at one point when I was very sick if I was going to die. Judy reassured her as well as she could.

I told him that I thought his surgeon was first-rate and that I would be thinking of him the next day and would see him soon. He thanked me and we said good night.

When I saw his surgeon late the next day and

eagerly asked him how it had gone, he told me that Barnes was dead. He had died at 6 p.m., an hour after the operation was over, the victim of a massive heart attack.

I could understand Barnes's death medically. I knew the circumstances and I understood the physiology and the anatomy. Yet it was a tremendous jolt. Two things about it occurred to me immediately. The first was that there was something too premeditated about it. He was executed. One evening he was a warm, vibrant, anxious, responsive human being, and the next evening, after voluntary human intervention, he was a corpse. He had not died on his own. Some freak of nature or spontaneous contortion of his own physiology had not killed him. He had died, more or less, at the hands of other men. The nurses sent his few belongings from the ward to his wife, as jailers might to the widow of a man executed.

The other unnerving thing about his death was that it was to some degree ordained by his own decisions. His heart was rotten and he would have died within the next few years in any event, but he was a physician and he knew about tests that could define his degree of disease and operations that could perhaps delay the inevitable. He chose those tests and elected the operation and in so doing he had himself killed. Knowingly, he took a reasoned risk, with the result that his two-year-old would never have the opportunity to remember his father as he might have otherwise. I find that sad and unsettling. Above all, I identify with Barnes's death because I was almost there.

By all yardsticks I had been very close to death at my first operation, yet I knew nothing of it. I had literally been put to sleep, dispatched to a painless never-never land, where hemorrhage and death benefits, love and grieving, religion and burial seem to make no difference. I was far from the battle, oblivious, tranquil. My family, I know, went through agony during the seven long hours I was on the operating table. I floated somewhere suspended, immune to the anxiety, ignorant even of the struggle. Barnes, as I see it, stayed there. I don't know if Barnes had a God or an afterlife to ransom him from that oblivion, but if he didn't his fate, his infinity was comfortable. His wife, his mother, and his children, it seems to me, had a much more difficult and sorrowful task ahead of them than did the slumbering Barnes.

I am glad that I came back to life after my surgery, but many times in the months of illness, in pain, in nausea, in fits of anxiety, in depression, poisoned by chemicals, burned by radiation, arm strapped to chest, chest festering, I recalled the tranquillity of anesthesia and longed for it. Barnes could have died a worse death.

CHAPTER
5

Revival

Social life in the hospital was very different from social life on the outside. Since I was always there and available, people could come and visit at any time. And yet I was still ill and didn't always feel like having visitors. The result was a continuous back-and-forth between me and the outside world, with Judy and my family often serving as intermediaries. Friends whom I might have expected to come regularly never showed up at all, while others, from whom I would not have expected a visit, spent extended periods of time with me. It was a new society.

Among the most welcome visitors was Mitch Mills. Although I was a resident of his floor and technically a patient on his service, the doctors who were caring for me now were the plastic surgeons. Dr. Mills's residents never even made rounds on me, yet once or twice a week Dr. Mills himself came by to see how I was doing. His visits were not only thoughtful but encouraging. We talked about his impending retirement from the Navy and what it would be like for him to begin private practice in middle life. We discussed the book I had written and problems with medical education. We chatted about his family and mine. The very ordinariness of our conversation was salutary for me. He didn't treat me as a patient with one arm sewn to a festering chest; he talked to me as a colleague and a friend, and this helped boost my image of myself immeasurably.

Dr. Mills had an uncanny way of showing up when I was most depressed and in despair that my latest strange surgery would never succeed. Later I discovered that the nurses on the floor kept him apprised of my situation and that he made a point of visiting when I was down.

One day he talked about a new hospital that the Navy was constructing next to the Tower Building. Work was already well under way for the complex of buildings that would replace the aging structures that housed the National Naval Medical Center as Dr. Mills and I knew it. As we talked, the bulldozers were excavating several acres of land, three stories deep, next door to us. "I have a very odd feeling about that hole in the ground," Dr. Mills told me.

"Why is that?" I inquired.

"I will die in that hole," he said simply.

I was taken aback. What could he possibly be talking about? He was in the prime of life, a surgeon among surgeons, on the verge of a second career opening chests and healing hearts.

"When I leave the Navy I will practice in this area. When I get sick I will come to the Naval Hospital, and when I die I will most likely die here. Those bulldozers and cranes are constructing the building I will die in. I can feel it."

The two of us sat quietly in that sunny room for a brief moment. He was robust and commanding in his lab coat, a study of a surgeon in his element. I was bandaged and dilapidated—and yet both of us had death on our minds. He was not immune from those thoughts, he seemed to be telling me. Mortality is with all of us—even the surgeon, who can seem invincible in the hospital setting. The surgical bravado and command promote an aura of omnipotence that can leave the patient—who is already painfully aware of his own frailty—feeling at a greater distance from health and strength. Yet here was a surgeon who was thoughtful and candid enough to share with me a little of his own anguish. To worry about death is human, he seemed to be saying . . . it is a problem for the surgeon as well as the patient.

When he left my room that afternoon, I felt strengthened.

After my first hospitalization, Judy and I had joined the Cedar Lane Unitarian Church in Bethesda. Ken MacLean, the minister there, had become our good friend, and now that I was back in the hospital, he was a regular late-night caller. Busy as Ken was with his many responsibilities, he seemed to enjoy after-hour sessions as did I. Frequently arriving long after the last visitor had left, he would bully and cajole his way past the nurses, who eventually accepted him without protest.

We talked about many things, including our families, illness, football, church politics, and writing. He was particularly interested in doctoring. I, of course, had many opinions about that subject and we spent time discussing holism, humanism, bedside manner, and the laying on of hands. He served on a committee at the National Institutes of Health charged with reviewing the ethics of proposed research on human subjects. He was intrigued with the gray zone between science and humanism. I suspect he had some of the same concern about religion, questioning the balance between the spiritual and the material.

There was one topic I raised with Ken that I discussed only vaguely with other people—my death. While I did not seem to be as ill now as I had been when my principal illness was cancer, I was aware of the treacherous nature of my open chest. The dangers of the skin transplant and recurrent infection kept me regularly in touch with the grimmest possibilities. Yet I was supposed to be curable and team spirit seemed to demand that I be bullish in my attitude toward recovery.

Still, I thought a lot about death and, more particularly, about the mechanics of dying. One night I unloaded on Ken. "Where *do* you get buried? How would *I* get buried? What's involved in a funeral or a memorial service? Who arranges all that and what should I do about it?"

Ken did a superb job of sorting out my tangle of questions and emotions. I was most troubled about where to be buried, a perplexing problem for someone who might die so young. My immediate family was alive to a person. Moreover, we were mobile Americans with no formal graveyard or family homestead. My grandparents had been buried in a variety of places with which I had no identification. The idea of being stuck in the ground at some arbitrary location and being left all alone gave me spasms of loneliness every time I thought about it.

I felt unburdened just to be able to tell someone about it. Ken assured me that if I died he would help coordinate the details. It was heartening to know that he would perform a memorial service for me at Cedar Lane. I even found myself imagining what the service might be like, who might be there, and what would be said. The whole topic was terribly morbid but I felt better for having talked about it.

By the late fall things had begun to improve. Dr. Colgan had reimplanted the chest flap at surgery and, at last, it seemed to be taking. The amount of infection had decreased and I began to gain weight and feel stronger. At first I was allowed home for an occasional evening, and then I was encouraged to take some overnights. In December, Dr. Colgan scheduled a date to detach my arm from the graft on the presumption that it was secure enough in its blood supply to maintain itself in place.

Before that, however, something else happened to raise my spirits. For more than three years I had been working on the manuscript of *White Coat, Clenched Fist*. Between bouts of illness I had finally finished the text and now the book was due to be published. Macmillan, the publisher, had agreed to sponsor a publication party and we had arranged to hold it at a downtown Washington bookstore. When the date arrived in December 1976, my arm was still sewn to my chest but we decided to go ahead with the celebration anyway since everything had been arranged.

It was a great party, just the tonic for a badly bruised ego. Droves of friends and acquaintances attended. The setting was congenial, the wine flowed freely, and the books sold briskly. I sat at a prim little desk with a single rose in a bud vase and greeted all comers. My inscriptions were in a chicken scratch, given the immobility of my arm, but I signed away nonetheless, triumphantly, defiantly.

It was a lovely evening, another celebration of life over death. I think Judy and Mom and Dad enjoyed it almost as much as I did and for the same reasons. Afterwards we returned to Mom and Dad's house with some friends for a late supper. We were exhausted and elated.

During the last weeks before I finally had my arm detached, I spent more and more time at home. Only then did I fully realize what four solid months in the hospital had done to distort my life. Coming home, for instance, meant eating meals with people instead of hunkering down alone in my hospital room watching television or thumbing through a magazine. Eating with others, it turned out, did wonders for my appetite. Coming home also meant the constant presence, pleasures, pressures, joys, and perils of living with two small children. That included companionship, fights at bedtime, hassles at mealtime, chuckles and surprises almost anytime. It meant being husband and friend to Judy regularly, not on an agenda defined by hospital visits and telephone calls. It meant sharing a bed, a fearsome experience since I was still bandaged, tender, and immobile and Judy is a restless though sound sleeper. Nonetheless, home was a joy after the hospital routine. I loved it all the more for the comparison I had the dubious pleasure of being able to make.

Every morning Judy stripped me of my old bandages and, after my shower, applied the new ones. The process was laborious, requiring half an hour even with good preparation. The actual application of the dressing varied little from what went on at the hospital but the scene at home was quite different.

Perforce, Caitlin and Meghan frequently attended the dressing ceremonies and enjoyed them thoroughly. Meghan was generally distracting, climbing on and off the bed and asking if this or that hurt. My belly button was a particular point of concern for her. Daily she reminded me that I was lucky to have it in place, an observation with which I could not disagree. A favorite pastime of hers was taking a roll of tape and bandaging as much of herself as she could. Massive wraps of tape over her feigned wounds somehow gave her gratification or a sense of identity with her father and she would often wear the bandages until they fell off.

Caitlin, on the other hand, was not big enough to climb on the bed. She was approaching her first birthday and could walk around the edge of the bed holding on to the bed sheets. She amused herself trying to pilfer forceps, gauze pads, scissors, or whatever she could get her hands on. When that failed she attacked the trash basket, tipping it over and entertaining herself by chewing on the foulest bandages she could find. The humor in our dressing ritual was not always apparent to me and Judy at the time. We frequently finished with Judy chasing the kids out of the room and me crawling around the floor angrily collecting utensils and wrappers that had been dispersed by Caitlin. Judy proved to be dexterous with the dressings, but both of us had to learn new skills of patience to carry out our daily routine.

In mid-December, I went to the operating room

for the last time to have my arm detached from my chest and returned to its normal position. Late in the afternoon on the day following surgery, Meghan and Judy were present in the hospital when Dr. Colgan came to change my dressing. Meghan, then almost five years old, had closely followed the plastic-surgical proceedings. The skin flap, obviously, had been a much more tangible evidence of disease to her than the invisible tumor. Furthermore, she had firmly grasped the idea that its dismantling was tantamount to the recovery of Daddy's health. So when Dr. Colgan removed the bandages she immediately asked to examine my arm and chest to make sure that there was no flap lurking anywhere. She was delighted with the results and as elated as if she had performed the surgery herself. "Daddy, I used to think you were going to die," she announced airily, "but now I know you are going to be better." During almost two years of illness Meghan had never before confronted me with her ultimate fear. Now that the skin flap was gone she seemed to be sufficiently relieved so that she could talk about it.

Dr. Colgan, sensitive as always, said that she was sure there were times when I thought I was going to die. I agreed and left it that I was glad to be alive and didn't plan to die now. We were all relieved that the long battle with infection and transplantation seemed to be over. Of us all, though, Meghan was particularly delighted and showed it.

My arm really didn't want to work. As pleased as I was to have it back in action, it wasn't really back. Four months of immobility had left me with very little motion at the elbow and the shoulder. I had so looked forward to feeding myself again with the accuracy that would only come from my right hand. I had anticipated good rigorous teeth brushings and being able once again to write simply and clearly. As it turned out, my newly liberated arm couldn't get a fork or toothbrush as far as my mouth and writing by hand, while possible, was terribly shaky.

The prescription for these problems was physical therapy, or PT, as it is known in hospital lingo. I had hopes that this would mean hot packs, massages, and whirlpool baths. I knew that was how the Washington Redskins took care of their joint and bone injuries and I was hoping to get some of the same treatment. The Naval Hospital PT Department had all of those therapies available, but they weren't for me. The routine recommended for my frozen joints was far less subtle or pleasurable than any of those treatments. While it went by more sophisticated names, what was in store for me was essentially the rack—regularly administered doses of painful stretching. The physical therapists, a fleet of good-looking ladies in tight white outfits, had a practical approach to their work. Affable and, of necessity, tough, every one of them approached my joints with crisp efficiency. At each visit they would spend twenty minutes levering, prying, and stretching my arm and shoulder in spite of groans, grimaces, and gnashing of teeth on my part. At the end of the abuse they would produce a goniometer (the name alone almost killed me) to measure my angles of movement. Slowly, over a period of several months, their tactics worked and I retrieved much of the motion I had lost, although there were moments in the midst of my stretching when I doubted that the recaptured ability to brush my teeth was worth it.

In spite of its shaky start, Dr. Colgan's skin graft finally worked. It stayed cemented down as it was supposed to and it fared well with its own blood supply developed at the peripheries even after the supportive arm was detached. Small areas of infection remained under the flap which necessitated wearing cumbersome bandages for almost a year, but slowly the infection dried up.

With the success of the flap, my weight and general well-being improved quickly, so that I could return to work shortly after leaving the hospital for the last time. For the first month I gingerly divided my days between the National Health Service Corps and physical therapy, slowly and happily phasing out the latter in favor of the former. Before long I was appointed Chief Medical Officer of the National Health Service Corps, assuming clinical responsibility for the program's practitioners across the country who were working as I had in Santa Fe. Once again the harness of work—the companionship, concerns, and responsibilities—felt very good. The obsessive focus on one's self and one's fate which periods of non-working sickness seem to invite was happily slipping behind me. The bustle and activity of the outside world were far preferable to the forced introspection of the patient, laying to rest any romantic notions that I had entertained earlier about the reflective luxury of sickness or the marvelous egocentrism of the patient. It was wonderful to be back on my feet and I was quite content never to be a patient again.

My sense of doctoring, I found, had been significantly changed by all that had happened. From medical school on I believed that medicine was something finite and specific, a marathon multiple-choice test in which, as physician, I was continually struggling to discover the correct diagnosis and match it to the right treatment. The greater the degree of accuracy I could bring to bear on my continuous skirmishes with disease, the better physician I would be. That had certainly been the emphasis of my disease-oriented medical training and residency. While I still appreciate accuracy and precision, my illness forcefully broadened my expectations of doctoring. A good physician was one who saw the patient as a whole person, a complex human being, rather than a series of organ systems in various states of repair. This was not an argument against knowledge or even specialization, but rather a recognition once and for all that good physicians are something more than Midas muffler dealers. Generalist or specialist, family practitioner or plastic surgeon, a good doctor needs to love his patients at least a little bit. He needs some curiosity, a touch of fervor, a belief that most people are good and worth knowing. Of course, no practitioner likes—let alone loves—all of his patients, and pure technicians function perfectly well in certain areas of medicine, but good patient care requires a sense of loving. If I had any doubts about that before being sick, I have none now.

As a patient, I felt that affection from Dr. Mills and Dr. Colgan and many others. There were as well nurses and corpsmen—particularly the corpsmen who spent so much time with me—who conveyed that same sense of completeness in their care. But there were others who did not. At one point while my arm was tied up, I visited the Plastic Surgery Clinic to be examined by the department's staff. One of the senior physicians who had seen me occasionally before started lecturing Dr. Colgan and others within earshot—including me—about what a great "case" I was. "This," he said, referring to me lying on a stretcher, "is simply a wonderful case. When the students are here, we never get a case like this, and now that the students are gone, here it is!" I felt belittled, cheapened. In medical school we had been admonished time and again never to call patients "cases." That was basic. Now it was happening to me and it *did* feel awful. "This case demonstrates a dozen surgical principles," he continued. "Most important, it represents a challenge. There's no way we can save this chest wall without our best work. Damned shame the students aren't here."

It really took being a patient to learn that the modern medical center is not an easy place in which to practice medicine warmly. The teams of doctors, all with a partial stake in the patient, the omnipresence of machinery, lab tests, and special procedures located hither and yon around the hospital, all promote an impersonality that can make connectedness almost impossible. Today's typical hospital bedside is not what usually comes to mind when we think of "bedside manner." A physician—or a nurse or a lab tech—has to be committed in principle and diligent in practice in order to overcome the natural anomie of the big hospital. From day to day, from shift to shift, from procedure to procedure, that didn't always happen and sometimes I was left feeling angry at my caretakers as well as at my disease. I came away from my hospitalization concerned about conveying this message to other physicians.

Age, I think, is on the side of sensitivity. The simple idealism of the incoming medical student is frequently overwhelmed and beaten down by the process of medical education. The student is taught, system by system, to be a technician. One week he is a kidney specialist, the next a pediatric surgeon, followed by a stint as a dermatologist, and so forth. This process makes it easy to lose sight of the human being. Unfortunately, all too often this becomes a permanent transformation.

It is a strange but unavoidable quirk in our system that those of us who become doctors are educated and turned loose at a time in our life when personal disease and debility are least likely. I can remember as an intern being frankly surprised at how many people were sick. I came quickly to understand that the 5 to 10 percent of the Gross National Product that most nations spend on health care was not a frivolous addiction but a reflection of the fact that the human mechanism is imperfect and requires a good deal of attention along the way to keep it running as well as possible. Yet a full appreciation of this comes more from personal experience than it can from either book learning or clinical exposure. I cannot help but think that all physicians, as they age and experience more infirmities of their own, gain a greater understanding of patienthood and human frailty.

This point was dramatized for me recently when I tried to explain it in the course of a lecture to a group of medical students. "We are all patients," I began. "A few of us become physicians as well." I proceeded to develop the argument that we should not think of ourselves as an elite but rather as help-mates to our fellows, whose biology and pathology are, after all, the same as our own. I concluded by urging them to maintain a sense of humility as they pursued their profession, suggesting that this would make them better physicians. This all was said, I reflected later, at precisely the time when they were doing everything in their power to join the medical fraternity. They were slavishly memorizing every sinew of the body, incorporating vast quantities of soon-to-be-forgotten biochemical data, and looking feverishly for role models among the diagnostic wizards of the faculty. All in all, it was an unpropitious time for the students to receive my message. They were killing themselves trying to achieve membership in the club while I was trying to tell them the club wasn't all that exclusive.

When I finished lecturing, the audience responded with indifference. Why, one student wanted to know, was I "down on" medicine? If I didn't want to be a doctor, another suggested, why didn't I do something else? I found the experience discouraging, but it gave me some insight into the changes I had undergone. Age, time, and personal experience with disease can reestablish a sensitivity that has been ground under by the exigencies of the educational process and the early years in practice. I was very fortunate to be cared for by Dr. Mills, who was clearly in touch not only with my humanity but with his own.

At about the time I left the hospital a reporter from the Washington *Star* approached me to see if I would be willing to have her write a story about my illness. My book had just been published and she was particularly interested in linking my attitudes as a doctor to my experiences as a patient. After much discussion I decided to let her do the story, hoping it would help me codify my feelings about my illness and, perhaps, be helpful to others.

Several weeks later, as I walked down a Washington street, I was startled to see a picture of myself seated with Judy staring up at me from a newsstand. "How a Doctor Learned He Had Become a Patient" read the headline on page one of the *Star*. My first response at seeing the picture and the headline was embarrassment. Why, I found myself asking, had I been so immodest as to spread my story over the newspapers? After reading the account, however, I felt better, since the reporter had succeeded in capturing the personal and familial trials of the disease as well as conveying the message and the hope that cancer *can* be endured. At the least, it was a well-told, human tale and it promised to offer insight and encouragement to families with similar problems. While the reporter and I together had not broken any new ground in science reporting, she had told my story in gentle yet provocative terms.

The headline for the second installment, which appeared the following day, read: "Grateful Yet Bitter over Technology That Saved Him." In part, this section dealt with the paradoxes of my situation. While radiation therapy had certainly helped to save me, it had also damaged me. Even though plastic surgery promised to release me from the afteraffects of radiation, it had held me prisoner for many uncertain weeks. In spite of having received the best medical care available, it had all been an awful experience. Toward the end of the article the reporter quoted me as saying: "Although I received more care than the average patient, I still had a lot of aches and pains that weren't treated. I got this test and that procedure, but the doctors would never consider rubbing my back. Physicians tend to be trained as super subspecialists. If your symptom doesn't fall into a fairly narrow zone, they tend not to respond at all or to respond in pat ways. I am not suggesting that the average physician can give a half-hour massage to every patient, but simply that he has to be more sensitive to the simple problems that haven't been dealt with well." Only once in the two articles was the National Naval Medical Center mentioned and nowhere did I speak specifically of the individual doctors or staff members who had cared for me. My musings were intended as a general commentary on contemporary medicine.

Folks at the National Naval Medical Center didn't see it that way. When I returned to Tower Nine for my monthly outpatient visit shortly after the articles appeared, there was a noticeable chill. People who had called me "Fitz" were calling me "Dr. Mullan" or avoiding me altogether. A doctor I knew only slightly saw me in the elevator and said, "Man, did you stick it to this hospital in that exposé. Your doctors are really burning."

I felt an immediate spasm of guilt when he said that. All of a sudden I couldn't remember what I had said in the articles. Had I really named names or told tales? Had I been bitter and complaining, a thoughtless ingrate? I *was* appreciative of the care and attention I had been given. I *was* delighted to be alive and thankful for the weeks and months of care that I had received at the Naval Hospital.

I went home and immediately reread both articles line by line. To be sure, the story was not full of accolades for the doctors and nurses who had cared for me. On the other hand, the pieces were not intended as a testimonial to either the individuals or the technology involved in treating my cancer. If anything, the account was a straightforward statement of a physician's struggle with his own disease. That struggle involved a certain amount of medical agnosticism and ambivalence about the modern medical center, but those were the dramatis personae of my tale as I told it and as the *Star* reported it. It was not a story of specific doctors, nurses, or institutions.

I was satisfied that I had not slurred the good name of the National Naval Medical Center or its staff. Yet, as far as I could tell, the perception at the hospital was that I had. In the following weeks, on visits to the hospital, I asked a number of people what they felt about the article. Almost without exception, those I questioned responded that they understood what I was talking about and had taken it in context. But, they added, many other staff members were really steamed up about it. I asked to come to the weekly meeting of the Tower Nine staff to discuss the *Star* story in an effort to explain my position and better understand what people were feeling. My offer was declined. The weeks passed without anyone really telling me off. Slowly the incident slipped into the background, leaving, as far as I could surmise, wounds to heal in many quarters. I felt very bad about the situation but could find no

forum to express either my guilt at seeming unappreciative or my anger at being misunderstood.

Outside the hospital the response to the story was
quite different. I received dozens of letters and
phone calls thanking me for my candor in discussing
my cancer. Generally readers seemed to feel that not
only the story but the frankness with which it was
expressed spoke to their problems and fears dealing
with their own illnesses or those of family members.
The very items that upset the hospital staff seemed
to stimulate my outside correspondents the most.
Time and again people commented on the gap between technology and humanism or simply the
paucity of human touch and understanding amidst
the modern therapies for cancer and other illnesses. I
received several invitations from local cancer groups
to meet with them and discuss my experience—
which I did. Inevitably I received calls from Laetrile
and health-food fanatics who wanted to share with
me their views on cancer cures. One caller who
claimed to be a chemist wanted to market a com-
pound that he said would cure cancers, lumps, and
bumps of all types. He needed someone with a medical license to help him market his product. Although
he was adamant that he would never reveal the
chemical components of his substance to anyone, he
did offer me 20 percent of the proceeds if I would
help legitimize his business enterprise. I declined.

In all, I was stunned at the gap between the medical and the non-medical perceptions of my story. The
hospital staff, on the one hand, saw my case as an

exceptional cure due to good medicine and good care, and that is the story they expected to find in the newspaper article. When they discovered something different, they took exception. Laymen, on the other hand, saw me as surviving despite, not because of, the trials and risks of modern medical care. Since one reads much less about the latter circumstance than the former, they responded supportively to my even broaching the issue.

As I reread the *Star* story now from the distance of several years, I can recognize a sense of frustration with my entire disease experience that was focused by the articles on my hospital care. Certainly I had legitimate observations and complaints about hospital medicine but, at bottom, I was mad as hell at just plain being sick. That anger was felt by my former caretakers both in the criticisms I leveled at the system and in the compliments I failed to pay them.

Yet my perceptions as patient had a foundation in the reality of my experience. I had lived in both worlds—the world of the doctor and the world of the patient—and I was coming to understand better the varying perceptions of the same events. There was no simple right or wrong in the potentially contrary interpretations of doctors and patients about hospital medicine. Both were rooted in realities—different realities. The *Star* story captured me as a patient. It invited health professionals in general to think critically about the personal aspects of their practice and the systems (hospitals) in which they worked. That

I believed—and still believe—is an important message but, as it turns out, one that can generate a heated response. That is what I felt from the Naval Hospital staff and that is what made me so uncomfortable.

I was still struggling with my role as a doctor-patient.

My strength and stamina continued to improve, and within a matter of months I was working and traveling as if hospitals and illness and cancer had not been part of my recent past. In September 1977, I was appointed Director of the National Health Service Corps, an exciting challenge and a wonderfully satisfying personal achievement, given my long association with the program. The new job was particularly rewarding because day in and day out it said to me that in spite of my illness I could still pursue the goals that mattered to me professionally, politically, and personally.

Throughout this period I never encountered what other cancer patients have come to term "shunning." Many people who have had cancer report that their relationships with friends, co-workers, and employers change dramatically when their diagnosis is discovered. I have heard many tales about problems, ranging from pragmatic but ill-informed responses by employers ("Cancer patients are bad risks") to just plain squeamishness on the part of people who, irrationally, seem to fear contagion. These stories are frequent enough so that I don't doubt that they are a real and agonizing part of the lives of many people who are struggling with cancer. Yet, strangely, I did not experience any shunning. Perhaps it was because my colleagues and so many of my acquaintances were involved in medicine and less subject to occult or outlandish beliefs about cancer. Perhaps also it was because my employer was the federal government and my job security was not subject to superstition or whim. In any event, friends and colleagues were generally understanding, sympathetic, and even, at times, a bit incredulous. People were often amazed and delighted that I had been able to wrestle with the monster and end up on my feet.

Throughout my months of illness and recuperation I experienced countless acts of support and encouragement by individuals connected with every aspect of my life. It is impossible to measure the total force of this web of assistance, but I know with certainty it had much to do with my regaining my momentum. While there may have been individuals who were driven away from me by my illness, I had no awareness of it. What I remember and cherish are the people who commiserated with me, helped me, rooted for me, pinch-hit for me, and eventually cheered for me.

When we left Santa Fe, for instance, Joan Shandler, the mother of one of Meghan's friends, wrote and illustrated a book called *Meghan's Moving Book*. It acknowledged how hard it is to leave your old home but showed Meghan making new friends and having an exciting time in Washington. Meghan loved the book and still has it in her bookcase. Steve Cohen, my medical school roommate, and his artist wife, Gretchen, supported us in myriad ways. For a long period Gretchen wrote to us almost daily—wonderful, intimate, diverting letters that were really a daily gift. Gretchen had a Christmas tradition of printing a woodcut of her own creation with some theme from the year and sending it to friends. The cards were actually a present—beautiful, thoughtful, and personal. The first Christmas after my illness—the Christmas, in fact, when Caitlin was born—Gretchen's card was a rough-cut portrait of four figures, pensively intertwined, Judy, me, Steve, and Gretchen.

The acts of kindness seemed to rise up to meet every new bout of sickness. Eamon McGhee, an acquaintance from work, arrived at my hospital room one day carrying a bonsai cypress tree that he had grown himself. It was a magnificent gift that took me by surprise and left me slightly tearful. My good friend and typist, Pauline Lieberman, made me a bulky, one-armed terry-cloth bathrobe to accommodate the exigencies of plastic surgery. It gave me and everyone on Tower Nine a good laugh. And on and on . . .

And yet the disease—the experience of the disease—remains with me. It is an indelible and inescapable part of me. As with the war veteran, things are never the same. As a friend put it, a Vietnam veteran, "Even though you don't talk about it or even think about it much, you can never forget the corpses by the roadside, the smell of death, and your own fear. You may get back to a three-piece suit and put Vitalis on your hair but you've been somewhere else— somewhere else that will always remain a part of you."

Most tangibly, I was left with physical scars. I remember filling out driver's license and passport applications in earlier years and chuckling when I came to the part that asked for "distinguishing physical marks or scars." That section was for Scarface Willie, not for me. I was a corn-fed American youth and, outside of a few moles, I had no "distinguishing marks." Now all that was changed. The average government form wouldn't have enough space for me to describe the surgically wrought abnormalities over much of my body.

The most noticeable scar and the one I had to deal with first was the one on my right forearm where the skin graft had been supported for its many months of implantation. The scar itself consisted of a prominent symmetrical three-sided track that ran almost from my wrist to my elbow. There was no way of avoiding its visibility unless I were to wear a shirt buttoned to my wrist at all times, so it was easy enough to decide that I would show the scar without reservations. Over time I have become comfortable with it and consider it something of a battle decoration. It does invite questions from time to time which are not easily answered. When someone queries me, "Oh, did you break your arm?" it is not easy to give a straightforward answer. Children often ask what it is and I respond that it is a dinosaur bite—since everyone knows dinosaurs have square jaws.

I have found the scars on my chest and abdomen less easy to cope with. About the time I became ill, men had started to wear necklaces and pendants. I had developed a fondness for Pueblo Indian bead jewelry called *hishi* that was prevalent in New Mexico. After the various surgeries, I was left with an indented chest with scars and potholes from my neck to my waist. Instead of wearing necklaces, I dress in turtlenecks or tight-necked T-shirts. I have not really learned to feel comfortable about these scars in areas of the body that are so identified with "manhood." When I swim, I keep a T-shirt on and I avoid public showers or locker rooms. I thought I would overcome these reticences over time but I have not. So I live with a negotiated peace between vanity and practicality, wearing my assortment of shirts at all times and retiring my beads. Judy and the kids have gotten used to my unusual architecture even though one of them will still ask me occasionally to explain again how this or that dent came about. A woman friend went on at great length about finding scars sexy. She fingered the ridges on my forearm and assured me that the scars were beautiful. My guess is that her tastes are the exception and not the rule.

Though the scars are the most graphic reminder of the past, there are dozens of other ligatures that keep me tethered to the cancer experience. Behind every cough, cold, ache, and pain there lurks the ghost of seminoma. Every flight or two of stairs leaves a shortness of breath that is the ever-present calling card of the ordeal. Although I don't smoke and don't like smoking, I have never gone to the extent of putting "No Smoking" signs in my office. Yet no one at work smokes in my office. While I appreciate the thoughtfulness of my colleagues, it is a bitter-sweet acknowledgment that they know that my chest is troubled. The future itself is peppered with uncertainties which Judy and I both worry about. These include employability, insurability, complications, and aftereffects.

It would be unfair, however, to characterize everything left in the wake of the cancer as negative. At intervals throughout my illness friends have suggested that I would be a better person for the "experience." Comments like "You'll come out of this for the better" or "You'll be a far more understanding physician because of your experience" have been frequent. When I was sickest and most desperate, these pleasantries infuriated me. I didn't want to be sick and, whatever my shortcomings, I didn't think I needed cancer to "improve" them. With the passage of time I have mellowed in my feelings. I think that people often make platitudinous comments about calamitous situations because it helps them to rationalize the otherwise awful circumstances. But experience—all experience—does change the individual and surely my ordeal is no exception. From it, I know that I developed skills of patience and resilience that will stay with me in other crises. I think I have learned something about what it means to be elderly, since I have had to live with degrees of physical compromise and incapacity that were unknown to me before. Disease *is* a sober teacher that leaves its pupils wiser—if not always thankful—for the instruction.

The illness has been beneficial in another regard. The traumas, fears, and joys that Judy and I have undergone have left us with a set of sensitivities about illness and the young family. Through the operations and hospitalizations as well as the birth and rearing of the children, we have unwittingly gained a host of experiences relevant to what it is to be young, committed to a family, and faced with potentially terminal illness. We really had no sense of the uniqueness of these experiences or our desire to share them until a young woman we knew slightly was diagnosed as having a malignancy of her thyroid. Susan and her husband, Cliff, were acquaintances whose child was enrolled in the same nursery school as Meghan. We learned from mutual friends that the thyroid biopsy had proved cancerous and she was in a local hospital awaiting a major operation that would remove her thyroid and perhaps much of the tissue on one side of her neck. The day we heard about it Judy called Cliff and offered to visit even though we had really spent no time with them previously. Our offer was accepted and we arrived at the hospital not knowing what to expect.

We spent two enormously intense hours with Susan and Cliff at her hospital bed that evening. We talked about children and scarring, chemotherapy and radiation, death and single parenthood, love, patience, fury, and luck. So many of the troubling and painful questions that they were encountering for the first time, Judy and I had battled for many long months. We had slag heaps of experience to share with them that a team of surgeons, clergymen, parents, and counselors would be hard pressed to provide. And I use the term "slag heap" purposefully, since so much of our experience had previously seemed like giant mounds of useless rubble—a strip mine through our lives. Now, as we talked with Susan and Cliff, those experiences assumed a purpose, a new usefulness. We could share them and plow them back into the newly broken ground of our friends' troubles and perhaps help them.

We left the hospital late that night feeling very close to two people we had hardly known before. Our friendship has continued with a special intensity since that time. Susan has had her ups and downs, but our support is four-cornered and very effective for all of us.

Although we have made no efforts to advertise ourselves as "cancer counselors," a number of people in the immediate area have sought us out for advice and discussion when cancer problems have arisen in their lives. These sessions and the resultant friendships are always rich and intense because of the peculiar bonds of shared risk and experience. I think it helps, also, to be able to approach a cancer problem with knowledgeable people *outside of* the purely medical setting. It is tremendously useful to cancer patients or families to find people who can help them to sift and digest the medical facts from the perspective of home and community. The facts and interpretation provided in the hospital or the doctor's office are, of course, critical, but the setting, the emotions, and the speed of events in the clinical environment don't always allow for the information to be absorbed or integrated. Occasionally we have been able to help in that way. Judy is superb at drawing people out and putting them at ease, and as time goes by we both hope to be able to make ourselves available in this way more often. In addition to the succor we try to provide to others in such encounters, it is rewarding to us because it converts some of the pain that we have been through into a positive force. It takes the detritus of our own ordeal and reprocesses it as something that is useful and salving to others.

Recovery meant a return to many things—activities, instincts, and interests that had been suppressed or overwhelmed by sickness. Some things were changed irrevocably. I was still an avid basketball fan, but playing an all-out game of pickup ball was something I would never do again. I resumed my interest in other things in ways that were unaltered —my appetite, my urge to write, my sense of politics.

Many pieces of my life, though, were jarred by the experience in a way that left them different from what they might have been otherwise, including the long-term plans for our family that Judy and I shared. As our lives returned to normal, we reveled in two healthy lovable girls who kept our hands and our hearts full. In earlier years, though, we had thought about having a larger family and we had discussed many possibilities, including more children of our own, foster children, or adoption. Increasingly, both of us felt that adoption would be an exciting experience since there were so many children in the world without good homes and we had, after all, already added our own two to the world's burgeoning population.

After our cancer battle we still wanted another child. We debated up and down about it, wondering about our future and the permanence of my cure. Were we too old? Did we have the energy? Was it too risky? Were we being unfair to the girls? Even the medical questions had no firm answers. The specialists I consulted, including the oncologist, could not guarantee that the radiation and chemotherapy I had received had not been damaging to my reproductive system. The problem had never been systematically studied and they could only counsel us that further pregnancy was not without risks.

The question, really, was a simple one to state though a hard one to answer. We were moving into the latter part of our thirties and, had I not been ill, we would have had more children. Were we going to allow the shadow of a disease which still fell over us to alter our plans? We decided that the answer was no. We wanted another child and we decided on adoption because it made both medical and social sense to us. Our desire to share our family with a homeless child coupled with the unanswerable questions about the effect of chemotherapy pointed almost unarguably to adoption. We quickly became eager about the possibility, with Meghan picking up on our interest and becoming a strong and persistent lobbyist for the idea. One day when I returned from work, Meghan, then six, greeted me with the news that she and Mommy had an announcement. They had decided, she explained, that we were going to adopt a baby soon and it would be a boy since she and Caitlin needed a brother. She was wildly enthusiastic. To her the thought of a brother was like Christmas, getting a puppy, and going to the circus all rolled into one. We were touched and even a little startled by her eagerness to share her home and her life. For a long time she felt that the idea was hers and we did nothing to challenge her. Meghan even wheedled her sister's endorsement, though the two-year-old Caitlin had little idea of what was happening. It was good to have the family united behind the idea.

The realities were more difficult. A visit to the local public adoption agency supplied us with the information that there were so few infants for adoption that families with natural children or with significant illness or over thirty-five were ineligible even for consideration. We were eliminated on all counts and had to look elsewhere. Judy became an expert in the field, reading scads of literature and joining several local organizations that were devoted to adoption issues. We were open on the question of race and considered Korean and Vietnamese as well as Latin American adoptions. We collected dozens of stories along the way, including my favorite—that of a friend of ours who had arranged an Ecuadorian adoption and, because of the expense involved, was nominated by a group of parents-in-waiting to go to the orphanage and bring back four infants by herself. With a load of Pampers and the help of the flight attendants, she traveled home with four bassinets filled with babies identified by Magic Marker messages written on their torsos. Her experience with adoption, like many others we heard described, had worked out marvelously.

The problem with foreign adoptions was that they were cumbersome and fraught with bureaucratic details. Nonetheless, we decided to apply abroad since it seemed the most likely to succeed. To complete our application we had to obtain copies of our marriage license, birth certificates, and the children's birth certificates. These had to be notarized, verified, certified, and authenticated by a string of officials that stopped just short of the Pope.

Judy set up an adoption central, opening negotiations with the State Department, the Immigration and Naturalization Service, several consulates, and the states of New York, Florida, and Illinois. Additionally, she had to find a social service agency that would do a home study—a detailed family examination that would assure the world that we believed in Sesame Street and Fisher Price toys, didn't beat up on each other, and served three square meals a day.

Several weeks after our agency interview, while Judy was in the midst of transshipping all of our documents, we received a call from the social worker who had conducted our home study. Would we consider an older American child, she wanted to know. There was a three-year-old boy from another state whom they had been asked to assist in placing. She knew that we had been planning on an infant but wondered if we might consider Jason. She put us in touch with the out-of-state agency so that we could get more details to assist in our deliberations.

At first we were reluctant, fixed as we were on the idea of a baby. It occurred to us, though, that a three-year-old would fit between Meghan and Caitlin, leaving both of them undisturbed in their respective places. An American adoption, too, was appealing to us since it meant solving a problem closer to home. It was hard, very hard, to weigh the loss of babyhood in taking an older child into our home. To be sure, we would avoid numerous late-night feedings and mountains of dirty diapers, but we would also be taking on a child with someone else's early imprint on him and we had no idea what that would mean. Some psychiatrist friends counseled us that nothing was more important to a child's development than the first two years—years which would have been lost to us. That was an unsettling argument, but even it was inconclusive, since, if true, someone might have done a good job during Jason's first two years. Who could know? The problem was insoluable.

The more we talked about it, however, the better we liked the idea of Jason. The next move—and one I suppose we should have realized would be irrevocable—was to meet him. It was arranged through the social service agencies to bring him in from out of state for a get-together. I had never been party to such a weird interview. We met at a cafeteria, Jason and his social worker, our social worker and us. At first glimpse it was clear; he was a beautiful child. But conversation was a struggle. Under the best of circumstances three-year-olds aren't much at dinner-table chitchat. Add four nervous adults, exclude by prior agreement any reference to anybody's family, and you have the makings of a decidedly uncomfortable dinner party. One of the social workers put her salad dressing on her spinach and I spilled ketchup, while Jason munched methodically through a cheeseburger, responding to questions in monosyllables. We engaged in such revealing exchanges as "How's the cheeseburger?" "Okay." "How do you like the restaurant?" "All right."

Things loosened up after lunch. Judy and I took Jason for a walk and did some shopping. We talked about this and that and stole sidelong looks at him, measuring his stride, studying his face, his build, his expression . . . It is no normal task assessing a child, weighing another human being for an hour or two, trying to decide if you are willing to spend the rest of your life with him, rearing him, supporting him, loving him. His body was strong and he would be a good athlete. That pleased me. At the same time I noticed that he was slightly knock-kneed when he ran, and I didn't like that. Would we *not* love him because he was knock-kneed? Could we turn him down and send him back, like damaged goods, because his knees bent in slightly instead of out? That was obviously silly, but the situation was so strange and uncharted that I knew neither *what* to think nor what to think *about* what I thought. Although I had been trained as a pediatrician and Judy as a social worker, nowhere had we been taught how to choose a child to take home.

After the walk, Judy and I had a chance to talk alone. We agreed that he was a lovely child, strong, handsome, and movingly brave in the face of what must have been an infinitely more bewildering situation for him than it was for us. We wanted to go ahead with the next step, which was to have Jason come home to meet the girls. When we arrived with Jason later that afternoon, Meghan and Caitlin were at a high pitch of excitement. They gave him a tour of the house that only a real estate agent might get. They showed him their toys, tested the TV several times, worked the swings in the yard, and ended up in the sandbox. We watched from a distance, trying to guess the chemistry of the trio. They certainly got on well that afternoon, but who knew what that meant for five years, twenty-five years, or a lifetime.

When Jason and the social worker got ready to leave at the end of the afternoon, I asked him ingenuously if he might like to come back to live with us for a while. The visit had gone so very well and there were warm feelings all around. He thought for a moment, scratched his head, and answered bluntly, "No." He had spunk—he wasn't going to be had easily. Whatever he understood about what was happening to him, he had his pride and his sense of his past and he wasn't going to throw all that over for a cheeseburger and an afternoon in a sandbox.

We respected Jason for his grittiness and our hearts went out to him, but the decision was going to have to be ours. Would we take this beautiful, abandoned colt and try to make him ours? Would we struggle to make him more like us and us like him, or would we look elsewhere for a different child, a younger child, a baby as yet unborn? The agency needed to know our decision quickly. We had only two days to sort out our feelings about Jason and ourselves, a short time by any measure to make what was obviously a lifelong decision. On the other hand, we really didn't have a lot of data to sift and weigh. Basically, we had the fact that Jason was a splendid, lovable, intelligent child whom we all liked immediately set against a series of unanswerable questions about his future. We spent two difficult days and nights wondering what to do . . . and in the end we concluded that it was a decision that had to be taken on faith—not, indeed, unlike biological birth. Any sort of child rearing involves risks and, in ways, we knew more about Jason than we would have known about an unborn child, somebody else's or our own. Meghan and Caitlin wanted him, we wanted him: we said yes.

It was a long drive to pick up Jason, but we took the kids as well as a portable party which Judy had arranged. The girls both had a small present for Jason and everybody got a new pair of pajamas. On the desk in the social worker's office we ate chocolate cake with plastic forks off plates that said "Happy Day." Jason was excited and tickled by all the attention. He seemed eager for his new life, his new home and sisters. He brought two cartons with him, one containing clothes and the other a little boy's bric-a-brac—two cars (one missing its wheels), a single drumstick, several rubber balls, three Golden Books, and a well-used teddy bear. We stopped in the parking lot and had the social worker take our first family picture. Before we had driven ten minutes on the way home the kids were all asleep from exhaustion and elation.

Jason was a wonderful addition to our family. The girls worked hard at making the adoption a reality and were probably more important to the process than were Judy and I. It felt good to share our home and to have a son, and many of the unanswerables about adoption were answered promptly because Jason was who he was—and is. We quickly came to love him.

One of my concerns then was one which Jason

could not answer—what a recurrence of my cancer would mean to him. We had worked hard to give him a home, but what would it mean for this game three-year-old who had already lost one family if I should suddenly become ill or, possibly, die? I mulled this problem before and after the adoption, with, obviously, no answer. After all the worry, it seemed to us that we should seize the day and live on in the best way that we could. Jason became another affirmation of life for us. We adopted his circumstance and he adopted ours, which included loving sisters, doting parents, and a risk—a risk that all five of us shared.

Cancer therapists talk in terms of a "five-year survival rate," by which they mean the number of patients with a given tumor who will live five years beyond the time of diagnosis. It is an arbitrary way of measuring human existence but useful for scoring the likelihood of escape from cancer. For many tumors, including seminoma, a five-year survival is about as close to a definition of a cure as anyone can come. In mid-March 1980, I tiptoed past the invisible line and into the future.

Well I remember sitting in a wheelchair in the Radiation Therapy Department one day during the first weeks of illness, waiting for treatment and wondering if by any quirk of luck I would become a "five-year survivor." It seemed so improbable then. I really didn't expect to be alive in 1980. Happily, it has come to pass and for that gift of life I am inexpressibly thankful. While I carry no warrantees with me and, in fact, would probably have difficulty getting a simple life insurance policy, I have had more than five years of living and growing since that first terrible discovery in the St. Vincent's Hospital X-ray Department. That is a richness that might never have been mine, as is the contemplation of the future. True, I am shadowed from time to time by the memories that I carry with me from the past and by the compromises which the illness has forced on me. Fear of recurrence will stay with me, as will the continued possibility of other medical complications. Nonetheless, it is great to be alive.

Late in my twenties I began to be bothered by birthdays as, little by little, they came to represent for me bench marks in the aging process. Each birthday meant one year less to live, one year further away from some vague ideal of youth. In fact, almost everybody I know complains about birthdays because they *are* reminders of the aging process—something most of us would rather ignore. It is as if we all carry around little purses with just so many coins in them and each birthday we are forced to give up one of our precious coppers, bringing us that much closer to an empty purse.

My feeling about birthdays, however, has changed dramatically since being ill. Each birthday is a victory—a small triumph over death and the oblivion that might have been. Each birthday is a celebration of the living, loving craziness of existence. For me, my birthday has become a thanksgiving event, since it means I have survived another year through physical and medical hazards. Unequivocally, that event is a celebration of life and not death.

CHAPTER
6

Taking Stock

If I had been born in any century prior to this one,
I would surely have died quickly from my cancer. It
is only in the last twenty years that the therapies that
allowed me to live have been available. In a strange
way, then, I have been born again—I am living a
second stage of my existence that might never have
been. At the very least I have the luxury of being
able to look back on illness and trying to make some
sense of it.

It is rare for someone in his thirties to become
seriously ill in America today. Sickness and death
were much more common for someone of that age in
earlier times before the advent of modern sanitation,
purified water, and antibiotics. Had I lived at the
end of the eighteenth century, three decades would
have been quite a reasonable life span. To have made

it out of infancy at all in those days was an accomplishment. I thought about Mozart and the incredible achievements of his thirty-five years. To be sure, schooling then was much abbreviated compared to what it is now, and young men and women married and went to work at a younger age. Although a thirty-two-year-old in 1775 would also have been at the height of his strength, illness and death for him would have been statistically far more likely than death for someone living in 1975. Death or the possibility of death for a thirty-two-year-old today is an uncommon occurrence and I was ill prepared for it.

During this time my role vis-à-vis my parents was in many ways inverted. While I was sick they both reached the birthdays that made them officially "senior citizens." Their good health and the passage of time had earned them more flexible schedules, the freedom to pursue academic and artistic interests, to travel, and to vacation with their grandchildren. They had reached a point where they were being rewarded for their age and accomplishments and were thoroughly enjoying it. At that very moment, however, they were involved in an unforeseen last fling with parenthood—a variant on the theme that Spock and Gesell had never written about. They were nurturing and protecting their adult son with an intensity that they had not experienced for almost thirty years. Daily they arranged and rearranged their schedules to make hospital visits. Mom made special brews of all sorts and brought them to the hospital or my home in an effort to promote weight gain. They drove me hundreds of repetitive miles around Washington for recreation (when that was all I could do), for doctors' appointments, for physical therapy, for anything that I needed.

And all of this took place at an age when the roles would normally have been reversed. I could have easily been pushing their wheelchairs, facilitating their medical appointments, or sitting in hospital corridors nervously awaiting the outcome of their surgery. Their strength and health were an enormous help to me. They developed a regular hospital routine for evenings—Mom carefully stowed a bottle of whiskey with my extra pajamas in the closet and she and Dad had cocktail hour with me regularly, drinking out of plastic cups with ginger ale from the Tower Nine galley for mixer. Late in the evening they would leave for dinner, famished but feeling warmed by a drink and a good visit. Mom writes poetry and often she would arrive with a folder full of verse that we would read and discuss. The many chores that Mom and Dad performed as well as their supportive presence made life much easier for me and for Judy. I did indeed feel nurtured by them and, as sick as I was and as downhearted as I became, I was continuously comforted by their strength and affection.

At the age of thirty-two I was not only a son but also a parent, a breadwinner, and a husband, roles which do not mix frequently or well with cancer. Everything that I had struggled to become was affected by my sickness. I felt particularly at sea with these problems since I knew no one else who had faced them at my age, nor was I aware of anything written on the subject. I had found no guides on "Fatherhood from the Hospital" or "Chemotherapy and Your Sex Life."

Meghan was just old enough to be aware of my illness from the time of its onset. To her great credit and my great relief she was concerned but loving and accepting through my ups and downs. In fact, I think I was far more critical of my performance as an ill father than she ever was. I had certain expectations of how I should perform as the father of a young daughter. When I was unable to deliver the goods, when I couldn't go swimming, when I couldn't lift her or chase her, or when I wept in her presence, I felt I had failed as a father. I think this perception was far more mine than hers and led to much useless angst on my part. The syndrome was all the worse because Meghan was my first child and I had developed some exacting and perhaps unrealistic notions about how loving, involved, and stern I would be. Even in good health it might have been difficult for me to be the kind of father I had conjured up in my own mind. Certainly, in ill health I had no hope of fulfilling my expectations.

In the early days of my illness, before Caitlin was born, Meghan and Judy spent a tremendous amount of time together and embarked on numerous projects of which I was not a part. This was especially true during my long recuperation from the first hospitalization. While I understood that Judy was protecting my limited energies by doing more than her share of child rearing and that Meghan, reasonably enough, was relying on the parent who she knew had the energy to engage her, I felt left out sometimes. I couldn't object, since I had no alternative, but at intervals I felt envious—and even jealous—of the intimacy they shared in many areas. Thinking about it one day, it occurred to me that their extraordinary closeness was a form of protection for both of them and not simply a club of which I was not a member. Since my life was still in the balance—a fact both of them appreciated in their different ways—they were busy building a cushion for themselves in case the worst came to pass. Mother and daughter knew they had each other no matter what happened and that was an important point of sustenance. This realization made me feel much better and far more accepting of their intimacy since I could appreciate their unspoken fear. My gradual return to health and the birth of Caitlin relaxed the intense mother-daughter intimacy of those months and returned me to a more active role in family projects.

Caitlin, of course, was born in the midst of our troubles and has known her daddy only with his scars. She did not live through a transition period from health to illness as Meghan did. For her the illness has been a given element of life and not something requiring adjustment. She has grown up affectionate and accepting, oblivious to the maelstrom from which she emerged. Jason, likewise, has inherited the history and vestiges of the cancer comfortably enough. They are simply another facet of his new family.

Life insurance, security planning, and retirement had never been part of my world. I really hadn't focused on the possibility of serious illness or, goodness knows, dying. Vaguely I imagined that "the system" would take care of me when my time came—which wouldn't be for decades anyway. Somehow I thought of life insurance as a scheme designed for rich executives with nothing better to do than buy themselves big financial cushions against the inevitable failure of their coronary blood vessels plugged by too many expense-account dinners and chauffeur-driven trips.

I am still no fan of the insurance industry. In fact, my very *un*insurability, due to cancer, increases my misgivings about the entire notion of private insurance. Yet the idea of security is far more vivid for me now than it ever was before. The sense of invulnerability that I carried with me as a healthy young person has been dismantled, leaving me with a much greater sense of personal wariness. Formerly my assumption of financial health was predicated on an absolute presumption of physical health. Now I am forcibly aware of how precarious a seeming state of well-being can actually be and how assumptions about a secure future can be converted overnight into a series of disturbing uncertainties.

After being sick, matters which had previously

been only perfunctory or peripheral concerns of mine became obsessions and led me into a snarl of unanswerable questions. How would the children's college education ever be paid for? What would tuition costs be in 1995? What were the merits of private vs. public education? What were the possibilities for scholarships, work-study programs, term-time jobs, etc.? I had to remind myself that Meghan was only struggling from nursery school into kindergarten. I spent time opening bank accounts for the kids and urging relatives to give them money instead of presents to put into the accounts. These modest savings provided a sense of security for me, even though their accumulated funds would hardly have paid for a year of day-care, let alone a year of college. All of a sudden the monthly mortgage payments became frightening. What if I couldn't meet them? Could we borrow money elsewhere or would we have to move? If we did have to sell and leave, what kind of housing could we afford?

Had necessity demanded, Judy could have resumed her career in social work. She and I spent time talking and worrying about that possibility. It was reassuring to know that she could make a living if need be, but Judy's pivotal role with the children and the household—a role that became more critical when I was ill—argued strongly against her return to work.

Through it all I didn't like *not* working. Part ego and part habit, work was terribly important to me. I felt rudderless staying at home day after day during my long recuperation, even though my physical condition necessitated going slow. For many people retirement proves a difficult transition after forty years in the workplace. For me, the prospect of retirement at the age of thirty-five was devastating, since I had neither inclination nor preparation to accept it. I was heavily invested in being a physician, and finding myself on the sidelines in slippers and a bathrobe worrying about sickness benefits, retirement plans, college tuition, and mortgage payments was painful. Work was wonderfully nourishing each time I returned to it, not only because it helped me reestablish my identity but because it provided me and the family with a sense of security for the future—a buffer I hadn't before sought or appreciated, but one that meant a great deal to me after having cancer.

Being a parent and being a breadwinner were not the only elements of my immediate identity that the illness challenged. Sickness of any major sort provides a head-on confrontation with a person's sense of his or her own sexuality. There is simply nothing sexy about vomiting, weight loss, surgery, or scars. I remember wondering, during my first hospitalization, if Judy would still find me attractive after all that was being done to me. After a few weeks of treatment and for many months thereafter I hardly cared, since I felt so physically wretched. In fact, for a long period I felt completely asexual. In much the same way that I lost track of my identity as a physician during my initial long hospitalization, I gradually became oblivious to my identity as a man. For a number of months sex was totally out of the question. Judy would cuddle and hold me from time to time, which felt good as nurturing but had nothing to do with eros. Nurses and female corpsmen would tend to my bandages and bathe me without any sense of sexuality on either side as far as I could tell. I didn't feel romantic, I didn't act romantic, and I wasn't treated romantically.

Recovery meant once again becoming something other than a neuter. I had to find out first of all if my body would function after months of surgery, chemotherapy, radiation, and physical wastage. Judy was a gentle and artful therapist, and little by little nursed me back to sexual health. Subsequent bouts of illness didn't do much for eros at our house either, but after the first, most debilitating round I felt more confident about my resilience. At every juncture Judy was patient yet solicitous, which was crucial in helping me reestablish my self-confidence. Thinned hair, scars, and bony ribs didn't seem to bother her—a fact that did a great deal to help me accept thinned hair, scars, and bony ribs.

Time and again over the years since that morning in the X-ray Department in Santa Fe, I have weighed my illness—sometimes philosophically, sometimes angrily, always in the belief that I would arrive at some point of indisputable logic, some wisdom that would explain once and for all exactly why I became ill. But the conclusion keeps changing. Like a kaleidoscope, every little turn of the chips leaves a different picture, the analysis altered. Sometimes I'm optimistic and even proud that I conquered cancer. There is an immodest swagger in my thinking. I licked the big C, I beat the cancer rap. Occasionally I am—crazy as it may seem—glad to have had the experience, since, like some daredevil, I have tested my limits and have some sense of what they are.

Frequently I am thankful to have simply survived and to be able to enjoy some more of life. I feel that way sometimes when Jason calls me "Daddy." How easy it would have been never to have known him or had him count me his Daddy. He has turned into a strikingly handsome boy with a passion for dirt bikes and a flair for sports.

Caitlin, now five, recently entered the Fourth of July Belly Flop Contest at our local swimming pool. She is a vivacious, intrepid child who keeps pet caterpillars, has fondled slugs and jellyfish, and prides herself on being the first one in the family to get into any body of water—no matter how cold or how murky. We squinted in the bright sun and watched as she pranced out to the end of the green diving board and grinned at us. She was missing one large front tooth, lost cleanly the year before in a playground tumble. She had labored successfully this year to convert her natural dive—a belly flop—into a real dive. The challenge in the belly flop contest was whether she could revert to her old ways. The competition would be keen since her category was all boys and girls eleven years old and younger. Fifty kids and half again as many parents watched as she sprang forward, arched her back, thrust her ample tummy forward, and spread her limbs. She hit with a magnificent, skin-slapping splash, her head still up and grinning mischievously. The crowd clapped and giggled its approval as Caitlin climbed out and waited for the judges (the lifeguards) to hold their scorecards aloft in mock-Olympic seriousness. When the last belly had been reddened and the results were announced, it was "Caitlin Mullan, eleven and under belly flop champion." Judy and I felt a thrill of delight at the news not only because of instinctive parental pride but because we were reminded again how lucky and unlikely was Caitlin's very existence.

A little sickness, though, or physical limitations due to my chest not working well will call forth a whole set of negative emotions. It is still easy to become bitter and feel cheated. Since there is nothing tangible to get angry at, I find myself becoming depressed and endlessly imagining my internal anatomy and its shortcomings. In my mind, I travel the two hapless segments of my severed phrenic nerve and speculate about their being rejoined—a surgical impossibility. I visit my heart and do damage assessment. I scour the corners of my chest cavity looking for tumor hideouts. The obsessional inventory does me no good physically or mentally, but it goes on anyway.

I think repeatedly about the operations I have undergone—particularly the first one. I wonder what if the biopsy had gone well and there had been no bleeding and no thoracotomy? What if, what if . . . ? Like a Monday-morning quarterback, I run and rerun the plays in my mind, fretting over a dropped pass and a missed block. During the hospitalization to rebuild my chest, particularly, I spent endless frustrated hours wallowing in these thoughts. But even now, at this distance, the possibility that things might have gone better and the results might have been more benign has an allure that I cannot avoid. This is especially preoccupying when I am feeling sorry for myself for one reason or another.

Part of me always wants to challenge my limitations as if to prove that they don't really exist. After a lot of work, I finally ran a half mile this year, a relatively trifling distance, but a long way for my chest. I dislike climbing stairs because I easily become short of breath, but in the last two years I've climbed several New England mountains and felt elated about it. Succeeding in an athletic challenge reminds me that things could have been a lot worse and, after all, most of me is still here and functioning.

Now and again I encounter someone whose handicaps are more pronounced than mine, and my perspective shifts again. Watching a teenager whose legs were severely deformed from birth struggle down a hill, across a dock, and into a canoe gave me that kind of jolt. She walked with her muscled arms, her limp, atrophic legs dragging behind her. Once in the canoe, she sat patiently waiting for her companions, who had disappeared up the hill on some mission of their own. She drifted aimlessly around the dock, paddling occasionally, for half an hour, captive of the canoe. Easy movement was a privilege she had never enjoyed. When her friends returned she asked them what took so long and they offered a casual excuse. She didn't protest, apparently accustomed to periods of waiting while the mobile world circulated about her. For a teenager subject to demands of conformity and the rigors of peer pressure, her deformity must be pure torture. If acne is a curse for the average adolescent, how does a fifteen-year-old deal with stunted legs and rippling biceps? She seemed pleasantly resigned to make the most out of her canoe ride and out of her life. Watching as she hauled herself around the dock without embarrassment, I reflected on my own modesty, wearing a T-shirt to cover my chest when I swam. Embarrassment is relative, she seemed to say. She did what she needed to do to get around, and if anyone wanted to blush or feel squeamish, that was their business.

Then, too, I know a blind woman who is a schoolteacher. She works a regular schedule, is married, articulate, and entirely open about her handicap. She has groups of her students spend "blind days" with her during which they don tight blindfolds in the morning and keep them in place until evening, functioning as well as they can with the assistance of their "sighted" classmates. I observed the teacher and a half dozen twelve-year-olds struggle through a cafeteria line at lunch. She coached and coaxed them at every stop, stoking them with various tips and tricks of the trade. While she was by no means complacent about her blindness, the teacher accepted it and used it to instruct young people who, for the moment, had no handicaps. They were learning precious lessons, I thought—ones on which I could have used more instruction along the way.

Observing the teacher as well as the girl in the canoe, I was impressed with the grittiness of the human spirit and felt a bit sheepish about my own complaints.

I now realize that I will never have a single conclusion about my cancer. Perhaps it was naïve to have ever thought that I would. Even as I write about it I can feel a kind of terminal ambivalence about the entire experience. Though I would never have chosen to have cancer, it is part of me and therefore something that I can't hate, deny, or discard. Like a lame leg or a blind eye, it is with me for the rest of my life. For better *and* for worse, I will live with it and quietly work and rework my personal history in an effort to accommodate it as much as possible.

The struggle to understand and make rational what happened has not been mine alone. Judy and the children, Mom and Dad have been affected and, in varying ways, have had their lives altered by all that happened. The kids, in particular, have grown up in the shadow of the cancer. Meghan asked me recently when my scars were going to go away. I explained to her, as indeed I had in the past, that they would always be there. "That can't be, Daddy!" She was incredulous. "You have done so well, the scars must be going away." She felt that everything *should* return to normal and I couldn't disagree with her. She found the permanent change in my physical reality hard to accept and so have I.

Being so close to the children, it is hard to assess the impact of my illness on them. At times I think it has given them a unique education, certainly an unusual and precocious one. Judy and I got a glimpse of this when our dog, Cinnamon, was run over and killed recently. Meghan was the most visibly moved by it. She called me at work and, between sobs, told me what had happened. I promised to come right home. When I got there the scene was an unhappy one. The children had been about to go for a walk when the accident happened. Cinnamon, ever friendly, had seen some other children across a busy street next to our house. Heedlessly, she sprinted across the macadam only to be struck by a car that never stopped. All of them saw it happen.

Cinnamon took about twenty minutes to die, trying to pull her crushed hindquarters out of the street with her still intact front legs. Cars slowed down; the school principal, driving by, stopped to help. Judy called the vet, who said there was nothing that could be done. Neighbors from across the street donated a blanket to put over the paralyzed, trembling puppy.

It was a terrible time for everyone there. For the kids it was especially painful. They had seen flies die on flypaper, perch expire on the bottom of a canoe, and numerous goldfish float lifeless to the top of our aquarium. But this was really death because Cinnamon had been one of the family. And they had observed every detail of her execution.

Meghan could not stop crying even long after I got home. Jason and Caitlin were upset too but spent more time worrying about what to do with Cinnamon. Where would Cinnamon "go"? Could we get another puppy soon? Judy and I felt sad, angry, and frustrated all at once but did the best we could to console them. Indeed, we had the problem of what to do with Cinnamon. Our house is on a small suburban plot without a rolling pasture or a friendly grove of trees where we could dig a grave for our pet. We had to bury her next to the house or not at all. Moreover, it was midwinter and the ground was frozen. I really wasn't sure if I could break the ground to dig a grave if I wanted to. My guess was that there was a county ordinance of some sort dictating where and how animals were to be buried.

So I called the county animal shelter. They offered me several options. First, they had the address of pet cemeteries around the county and they assured me the cemeteries did a good job. Second, if I was willing to transport the dead dog to the county animal shelter, they would dispose of it for me, free of charge, or keep the body until I had made cemetery arrangements. Third, they had the number of a lady who, for a price, would come and pick up the body and dispose of it herself. She was very efficient, they told me. As for any ordinances about burial, they were sure there were some rules governing it but they couldn't seem to find them. Their advice was simply to bury her deep and use some quicklime.

We chose the last alternative, although it meant rolling up our sleeves and getting involved in death and dirt in a way that I didn't relish. Cinnamon would remain close to us in death as she had been in life. It was getting dark and a light snow had started to fall. Jason and Caitlin and I picked a spot between our small wood pile and the driveway, not far from the side of the house. Meghan wouldn't participate but watched every move from her window. It turned out that the spade was equal to the frozen ground, and in twenty minutes we had dug a hole three feet deep, three feet long and three feet wide. Caitlin and Jason chattered the whole time, wondering why it had to be so deep, or just how Cinnamon would lie, or would she like it, or how it would feel with all that dirt around you. The dirt and the hole turned white with a dusting of snow and we had to turn on the car headlights in order to see where we were shoveling.

The neighbors who had supplied the blanket for Cinnamon's last comfort had also picked her up and put her in their garage after she had died. They explained that, three years before, their dog had been killed in the same spot and they understood what we were going through. Cinnamon was a stone-like weight in the black garbage bag which the three of us carried carefully back across the street. We lifted her caked, tepid body out of the garbage bag and put it in the hole. The kids were torn between looking the other way and studying every detail. They did a little of both while Meghan watched from her window. Standing in the light snow, we paused for a moment of silence for each of us to think about Cinnamon before we put the dirt on her grave. Then we sprinkled quicklime over the body and started to shove the dirt back in. "Poor Cinnamon," Jason offered, "she'll freeze to death out here." We packed the dirt down tight, turned off the car lights, put away the shovel and quicklime, and returned to the house feeling a bit better. Even Meghan seemed a little happier. That night Caitlin said to me, "Daddy, you almost died but you didn't." She hugged me and looked happy and a little smug. "I'm glad you didn't." She has repeated this theme frequently, saying things like "Cinnamon died but Daddy didn't."

Meghan was genuinely and deeply upset by Cinnamon's death in a way that surprised us. Her grief was so profound and so baleful that we wondered where it came from. Had years of holding back the tears given her cause to cry all the more when death really occurred? Was separation especially hard for her because she had spent so much time contemplating it? Or was she simply more straightforward about her feelings than anyone else?

Although that was some months ago, Cinnamon is still very much with us. When we see friends whom we haven't seen for some time, one of the children usually brings up Cinnamon's death. The tone now is matter-of-fact but the subject is never far from their minds. Pictures of Cinnamon hang on the bulletin board in the kitchen, where, willy-nilly, we spend a good deal of time. The other day Jason dropped a piece of food while eating dinner. "Cinnamon would eat that up right away," he commented with accuracy, "if we had a Cinnamon."

The TV screen focuses on a diner. It is twilight and the restaurant lights are out. A young man on the inside flips over a sign hanging on the glass door. The sign reads: CLOSED. He steps out of the door, locking it carefully behind him, throws his leather jacket over his shoulder, and ambles listlessly down the block. As he departs the announcer explains that he had planned to go to college but his father had died, leaving the family unprepared. Presumably the young man will spend his life doing odd jobs.

This vignette is a life insurance ad which would have meant little to me before my illness, but it troubles me greatly when I see it now. My first response is sadness—terrible sadness. The boy is Jason and he is a short-order cook because I failed him—because I died. That possibility is painfully sad. My next emotion is indignation. No, I say, it doesn't have to be that way. I know my kids will land on their feet. The ad has no right to threaten us. They shouldn't allow that kind of thing on TV. Finally, I settle into a review of all the reasons why the family would be all right if I died and, so doing, relieve the pain of the diner scenario.

The fear of loss—the anticipation of life that I will

miss—is perhaps the strongest emotion that I have regularly experienced, and it is evoked by many things. The children call it forth most predictably because I can visualize the future for them. The idea, for instance, of Meghan graduating from high school ten years hence without me is real and very upsetting. Other events are less foreseeable and therefore not as powerful in the melancholy they summon forth. But, over time, I have done a lot of grieving for the future on the chance that I might not be there. That is a strange way to spend time and emotion.

If I had died quickly in a car accident or in Vietnam or from some swift ailment, I would not have spent much time reflecting on what it was that I was losing. Having been confronted with death, however, over a long period of time, I have had the opportunity to examine all of its implications and penalties. That has not been easy. Often, especially when things look their glummest, I have wished for a speedy death—a death in a plane or a drowning or a car where there would have been only a few seconds of knowledge and contemplation. Speed seemed to be clean and merciful.

Why should the prospect of death be so punishing in itself? Why would I not accept as much life and pleasure as I could without being haunted by the possibility of death? The answer is that the ongoing experience with disease has made me stingier and more covetous of my presumed entitlement to life. In fact, the possibility of the loss of my life troubled me so that enjoying what I had proved difficult at times.

I had become a hoarder of life and, like anyone with a hoard, the possibility of its loss became more powerful than the joy of its possession.

Somewhere along the way I realized my predicament. A little good health, being able to eat again, and getting back to work helped a whole lot. The fun, the satisfaction, the chuckles that make up life are not finite. There are as many of them out there, I came to feel, as I could get hold of. The joy of a skill rekindled was often greater than what I remembered. This was true for eating Chinese food and oysters, swimming, mountain climbing, visiting New Mexico, and doing many of the things I had often taken for granted before. In many ways life had more flavor and more verve after my illness than before it.

In no way do I mean to recommend or endorse serious sickness, but living through it has, I think, left me with a fuller sense of life. This sense includes the inevitability of death attended by some quantity of pain and despair as well as the richness of life in the years that are ours. The predictable is not life and health but rather death. I say that not in any spirit of morosity but rather with a reinforced sense of the muscularity and mischief, the loyalty and generosity, the sensuality and humor that are ours for the time that we are here. The joy of Caitlin's birth and Jason's adoption, the warmth of family love, the satisfaction of my first book and this one, and a host of other daily events are sensations I might never have known. Those experiences confirm for me that, whatever its weight, life is good and worth having. I say that not only to those who are healthy and bored and to those who are sick and depressed, but also to myself, who suffers still from occasional bouts of hoarders' melancholy.

Sometimes in the bustle of rekindled life, amidst the demands, the distractions, and the fatigue, I forget how good those things really are and how easily they might not have been. That is a simple message and a happy one—and one that I am delighted to be able to share.